Missing Peace

Eleven Secrets to Restore Inner Harmony
with Your Food, Body, and Health

Melanie M. Jatsek, RD, LD

BALBOA.
PRESS
A DIVISION OF HAY HOUSE

Balboa Press books may be ordered through booksellers or by contacting:

Balboa Press
A Division of Hay House
1663 Liberty Drive
Bloomington, IN 47403
www.balboapress.com
1 (877) 407-4847

Because of the dynamic nature of the Internet, any web addresses or links contained in this book may have changed since publication and may no longer be valid. The views expressed in this work are solely those of the author and do not necessarily reflect the views of the publisher, and the publisher hereby disclaims any responsibility for them.

The author of this book does not dispense medical advice or prescribe the use of any technique as a form of treatment for physical, emotional, or medical problems without the advice of a physician, either directly or indirectly. The intent of the author is only to offer information of a general nature to help you in your quest for emotional and spiritual well-being. In the event you use any of the information in this book for yourself, which is your constitutional right, the author and the publisher assume no responsibility for your actions.

This book is a work of non-fiction. Unless otherwise noted, the author and the publisher make no explicit guarantees as to the accuracy of the information contained in this book and in some cases, names of people and places have been altered to protect their privacy.

Any people depicted in stock imagery provided by Getty Images are models, and such images are being used for illustrative purposes only. Certain stock imagery © Getty Images.

Print information available on the last page.

ISBN: 978-1-9822-1046-5 (sc)
ISBN: 978-1-9822-1047-2 (e)

Library of Congress Control Number: 2018909805

Balboa Press rev. date: 09/20/2018

To my mom and dad, MaryAnn and Ron Chura: Thank you for bringing me into this world, serving as my loving guides, and modeling true, unconditional love while showing me what it means to live with undying faith.

To my husband, Wayne: Thank you for sticking by my side as I explore life and discover my purpose. Your patience, love, and support give me the courage to express my highest self. I love you with all my heart.

> A man who as a physical being is always turned
> toward the outside, thinking that his happiness
> lies outside him, finally turns inward and
> discovers that the source is within him.
> —Soren Kierkegaard

Contents

Preface..ix

    How to Read and Use This Book..xiv

    Do-It-Yourself Shakes...xvi

Introduction..xxi

    Path to Peace..xxxvii

Chapter 1: Allowing...1

    Missing Peace #1: Seek No Further...2

Chapter 2: Anchoring...13

    Missing Peace #2: What You Resist, Persists.........................14

    Missing Peace #3: No Food Is Forbidden...............................23

Chapter 3: Trusting..31

    Missing Peace #4: What You Feed Your Body Most,

    It Will Crave..32

    Missing Peace #5: Return to Your Roots.................................54

Chapter 4: Craving...67

    Missing Peace #6: Awaken to the Source of Your

    Unsupportive Cravings...68

    Missing Peace #7: Imperfection Is Perfection.......................90

Chapter 5: Thinking and Believing 103
    Missing Peace #8: What You Think about, You
    Bring About 104
    Missing Peace #9: Choose Carefully the Words
    Following "I Am" 123

Chapter 6: Connecting 131
    Missing Peace #10: Live with the End in Mind 132
    Missing Peace #11: Connect to Your Inner Voice...................144

Closing 155
    Rest in Living Peace.. 155

Recipes 161
    Peace of Health Shakes..161
    Earthfood Powder 162

Appendix..171
    Earthfoods 171
    Functional Foods..176
    Product Recommendation List 177

Bibliography..179

Index 183

Preface

In September of 2015, I had an epiphany. And it was concerning the very book you are holding in your hands: *Missing Peace*. Boom! Just like that, the title flashed before my eyes. This was a true gift from my higher self.

I explored it a bit more and began to feel a strong urge to write a book that shared all of the pieces that people tend to ignore or miss when they set out to improve their health.

I got super inspired because I now had a platform to share my knowledge and passion with the world. It's what I've felt for years and the source of my frustration when friends, family, or clients would hop on the next diet. Instead of being supportive, I would shoot it down and become angry: angry at myself because I couldn't help them. At one time, I was them and knew deep down where this diet would lead them. They didn't need another diet; they needed a deeper understanding of themselves and their immense power. They needed to understand the missing pieces in their lives that were keeping them from achieving lasting peace with their food, body, and health. The peace that is their birthright.

I credit my inner voice—the voice of my higher self—for the countless gentle nudges to pick up my pen and write, and the frequent flashes of genius ideas that would eventually make up all of the missing peaces in this book. The process was simply perfect, like a well-rehearsed symphony. This voice would not let me rest. When I say this book was begging to be written, I mean that quite literally.

Part of this perfection included the right teachers appearing in my life at the right time, with the exact message that I needed to hear at the moment.

One particular month, I was really dragging my feet. I hadn't written a single word in nearly three weeks and was feeling quite awful about it. What was the source of this resistance? Was it fear? Complacency? Lack of belief in myself? Looking back, I'm certain it was a little of all three wrapped up into one, with a generous sprinkling of creative numbness.

I was going through a difficult time in my life, which caused me to question my spiritual beliefs. I went through the motions of meditation, contemplation, gratitude journaling, and all of my other daily rituals, but the feeling was missing. The spark that gave me hope was extinguished.

It wasn't until the personal challenges became so overwhelming that I experienced an emotional volcano. Spending three full days crying my eyes out and at times gasping for air, I repeatedly asked Divine energy for help. I clearly couldn't do this on my own.

The next day, I was running on the treadmill while listening to a Wayne Dyer podcast. He was interviewing a woman named Bronnie Ware, author of *The Top Five Regrets of the Dying*. She was a palliative care nurse who spent many hours with patients in their final days of life.

As you can imagine, she had some pretty heartfelt conversations with these individuals, and out of them came her book. Dyer asked her about the number one regret of those on their deathbed, to which she replied, "I wish I'd had the courage to live a life true to myself, not the life others expected of me."

Bronnie's statement hit me like a ton of bricks. I pictured lying on my deathbed, with only hours of life left. I imagined any and all regrets that could possibly surface during my final moments as I reflected back on my time on earth. The only regret that I could fathom was not writing this book. Why did the absolutely perfect book title appear out of nowhere? Why did I go through three years of hell with a binge-eating disorder? Surely this all had to come from somewhere. Then, I heard a voice as clear as if it came from a person standing next to me: Live as if today were your final day on this earth. From now on, Melanie, live without regret.

It was at that moment that I vowed to turn my years of pain into a solution for others. I had no choice, really, because failing to do so meant it would haunt me for the rest of my life. This tells me that something bigger than me is insisting this is my mission. And deep down inside, I know it is. I know for sure because when I step away from writing out of fear or playing small, I feel unsettled—a clear sign that I am disconnected and out of alignment with my calling.

Thank goodness I experienced that three-day emotional cleanse. It served to scrub all of the layers of excuses and bullshit that I had been feeding myself for why I wasn't good enough to write this book. It scrubbed and scoured until it reached my core, my soul, my essence. I am eternally grateful for the circumstances that brought me to this breaking point, for it exposed my inner light.

The concept of this book was born out of a burning desire to share my message with the world, to share the lessons I learned in hopes that it will help just one person. I've always said that if I can help change just one person's life for the better, I could die tomorrow at peace. This book is for that one person—you.

The book you are about to read is more of a journey. My voyage from a vicious disease called binge eating disorder to a life full of freedom, bliss, and health. Out of this journey came a solution. It's nothing you will find in any diet or nutrition book. In fact, you may not be ready for it.

This book is for the open-minded, the self-blamers who are sick and tired of the uphill struggle, the topsy-turvy, loop-de-loop battle with food and their health. It is for you, my friend; you know who you are. The one who feels lost and not quite sure where to turn. The one who awakens every morning in despair, believing that this is the best life has to offer. You have no idea how wrong you are.

We may have never met, but I love you. I was once you and managed to claw my way out of the dirt and grime of an unhealthy body and out-of-control mind, only to claim the one who was waiting for me to arrive. There she was, the real Melanie. The formless Melanie. The Melanie before the name, gender, labels, and occupation. When I finally stepped into her, a feeling of immediate peace washed over my body. I was home. Everything in my life got better: my health, my relationship with food, and my relationship with others.

This space is 100 percent pure Divine love. When I'm connected to the real me, I feel on purpose and on top of the world, like I can be, do, and have anything I want. In fact, I am in that place right this very moment as I write these words, a place of unconditional bliss and peace.

If you are reading this book, chances are you are missing the feeling of peace and well-being in your life. But consider this: In order to miss something, you must have had it at one point—even if just for a split-second. If you long for a state of harmony with your food, body, and health, this means you must know what it feels like to *be* in harmony. This book will teach you how to return to that good-feeling, peaceful place in a literal instant—because it never went anywhere.

If you have an open mind and are ready to learn more, please read on. If you don't know where else to turn, read on, because I promise you this experience will be like turning on the light switch in the dark room of your life.

How to Read and Use This Book

To get the most out of *Missing Peace*, I suggest you read it first in its entirety. Then, go back and read one lesson at a time, spending a full week contemplating the message and practicing the suggested Make Peace exercises at the end of each lesson.

Because this is the furthest thing from a diet book, I will not be offering you meal plans or lists of foods to avoid. Let's face it: You've been through that already, and it's no fun. Instead, I will be offering you simple Peace of Health shake recipes to try as you move through this journey and experience each Missing Peace.

Why a shake? About ten years ago, I went on the hunt for a simple breakfast that would pack the most nutrition possible in one container. I found my solution in a shake.

Some people ask, why not just eat the food instead? That's a fair question. If you think about it, though, how likely are you to sit down with a fork and eat a plate full of kale, avocado, berries, almond butter, turmeric root, and chia seeds for breakfast?

My Peace of Health shakes offer the best of both worlds: nutrition and convenience. All you need is a blender, a handful of ingredients, and five minutes. Each shake contains at least three servings of Earthfoods, which are whole, plant-based, nutrient-rich foods from the earth. They are powerful beyond measure and include vegetables, fruits, beans, nuts, seeds, herbs, spices, and other natural whole foods.

You will learn more about Earthfoods in Missing Peace #4: What You Feed Your Body Most, It Will Crave. In the meantime, a list of Earthfoods and all of the Peace of Health shake recipes can be found in the appendix.

One thing you will notice immediately about my Peace of Health shakes is that they are not sweet. Well, I should rephrase that; they do not taste sweet to people who have trained their taste buds to prefer sweeter foods. You will soon learn that sweetness is a trained preference, one that can be changed. The goal is to recalibrate your taste buds so that you begin to pick up the natural sweetness of the small amount of fruit in the shakes, without having to add sweetener or extra fruit.

You must be able to understand what it feels like to occupy a body that is healthy and energized. It's true that we don't know what we don't know, so if you've been walking around in a fog for the past two, three, or ten years, with aches, pains, and low energy, you'll have no way of knowing just how good you could be feeling.

Your health is important to me; therefore, I suggest very strongly that you drink one of the recommended Peace of Health shakes every day. It works best if you drink it for breakfast, as a positive way to begin your day and to set the tone for good food choices to follow.

Do-It-Yourself Shakes

If you prefer to create your own Peace of Health shake, here are five components you should include to ensure it is well-balanced and satisfying:

1. Liquid base: The best base for your shake is one that's low in sugar, without added artificial sweeteners like sucralose (Splenda) or aspartame. Choose water, coconut water, unsweetened green tea, unsweetened almond milk, cashew milk, coconut milk, or flax milk.

Amount per shake: 10–16 oz. (when adding avocado, use the upper amount).

2. Healthy protein: Protein is essential for balanced blood sugar. It also slows digestion and helps to keep you full so you eat less. Healthy protein sources include plant-based protein powder; bone broth protein powder; fresh ground nut or seed butter (almond, peanut, cashew, sunflower, etc.); tahini; or flax, hemp, or chia seeds. You could also whip up a batch of my Earthfood Powder, which is a homemade protein powder (see the recipe below). Note: Nuts, seeds, nut/seed butters, tahini, and Earthfood Powder also double as a healthy fat.

Amount per shake (pick one to two servings): One-half to one scoop plant-based or bone broth protein powder; 2 tbsp. Earthfood Powder; 1 tbsp. nut butter, seed butter, tahini, or flax/hemp/chia seeds; 2 tbsp. nuts or seeds (almonds, cashews, macadamia nuts, peanuts, pecans, pine nuts, pistachios, walnuts, pumpkin seeds, sunflower seeds).

3. Healthy fat: Most people forget to add healthy fat to their shake. Eating too little fat causes increased hunger and cravings, lowered metabolism, and weight gain (yes, weight gain). If you want to stay satisfied for hours, add a serving or two of healthy fat to your smoothie, such as fresh ground nut or seed butter (almond, peanut, cashew, sunflower, etc.); tahini; flax, hemp, or chia seeds; coconut oil or butter; medium-chain triglyceride (MCT) oil; avocado; or Earthfood Powder. Note: Nuts, seeds, nut/seed butters, tahini, and Earthfood Powder also double as a healthy protein.

Amount per shake (pick one to three servings): 1 tbsp. nut or seed butter; 2 tbsp. nuts or seeds (see Healthy Protein above for a list); 1 tbsp. tahini; 1 tbsp. chia, flax, or hemp seeds; ½–1 tbsp. coconut oil or butter; ½–1 tbsp. MCT oil; ½ (small) or ¼ (large) avocado.

4. Veggies and fruits: Boost the cleansing power of your shake with a couple servings of healthy carbohydrates, like spinach, kale or other greens, greens powder, carrots, beets, frozen cauliflower, berries, banana, apple, or pear. Fruits and veggies also offer a healthy dose of fiber, which can help prevent constipation. Bonus!

Amount per shake (pick one or two veggies and one fruit): 1 big handful of spinach, kale, or other green; 1 big handful of cabbage; 1 scoop greens powder; ½–1 cup carrots, beets, or frozen cauliflower; ½ cup canned pumpkin (not pumpkin pie filling); ½–1 cup fruit.

5. Functional foods: Functional foods are foods that have a potentially positive effect on health beyond basic nutrition. They are super easy to add to a shake. Functional foods include herbs and spices such as turmeric, ginger, cinnamon, cacao powder, maca powder, and matcha.

Amount per shake (pick 1–3 servings): 1 tbsp. cacao, fresh turmeric, ginger, or other herbs/spices; ½ tsp. matcha; ½–1 tsp. maca, cinnamon, powdered ginger, turmeric, or other herbs/spices.

For a thicker shake, add between a ¼–½ of a peeled and seeded avocado or use less liquid.

For a sweeter shake, try adding one of the following:

- a natural flavor enhancer, like a few dashes of ground cinnamon; a wedge of lemon, lime, or orange; a few sprigs of fresh mint; or a teaspoon of organic, pure vanilla, or peppermint extract
- ¼–½ cup more fruit
- up to 1 tsp. of raw honey, pure maple syrup, coconut nectar, or a pitted date

How to Make Your Own Coconut Milk

To a glass container with a tight-fitting lid, add one can (13.5 oz.) of organic, unsweetened, full-fat coconut milk plus four cans of water. Shake until combined. Refrigerate and use within four days.

Earthfood Powder
2 Earthfoods per servings ❤❤
Serving size: 2 tbsp.

1 cup raw pepitas (pumpkin seeds)
1 cup hemp hearts
1 cup milled flaxseed
1 tbsp. ground cinnamon
1 tbsp. raw cacao powder
1 tsp. sea salt
1 cup Bob's Red Mill Pea Protein Powder

Instructions:

Add pepitas through sea salt to a food processor or blender and process until seeds are broken down (about 1 minute). Pour contents into a large mixing bowl or container with lid and add pea protein, mixing/shaking until thoroughly combined. Store in airtight container in refrigerator or freezer.

Nutrition Facts per serving (2 tbsp.): Calories: 100; Total Fat: 7 g; Saturated Fat: 1 g; Sodium: 150 mg; Potassium: 0 mg; Total Carbohydrates: 3 g; Dietary Fiber: 3 g; Net Carbohydrates: 0 g; Sugar: 0 g; Protein: 8 g

Introduction

When I was a little girl, Popsicles and ice cream cones were something you ate when it was hot outside. There was nothing like a cool treat on a warm summer afternoon.

In our backyard stood a four-foot aboveground pool, the destination spot for all the neighborhood kids. During summer vacations, I spent nearly every day splashing, soaking, and floating in that pool. There was something about swimming that really revved up my appetite. When hunger struck, I would take a quick break, just enough time to dry off, run inside, and help myself to a fruit-on-the-bottom yogurt. I usually filled up halfway through and, without a second thought, placed the half-eaten container back in the refrigerator and walked away. No big deal; I had water to splash and friends to play with. Food was indeed secondary. Little did I know at the time that I was practicing what the Japanese call *hara hachi bu*: 80 percent full. Not stuffed but almost full. It never crossed my mind to finish the entire cup; after all, why would I? I was satisfied. Food was secondary.

Growing up, beef vegetable soup, homemade spaghetti sauce, and beef stroganoff stand out as dinnertime favorites. When dinner was over, I no longer thought about food. I never felt the need to clean my plate unless forced to by Mom and Dad, which became a daily ritual up until around junior high school. Leaving food on the plate was considered a sin; after all, there were starving children in China. But I could always count on Corky, our beloved cockapoo, to quietly take a few scraps out of my hands under the table. It was our little secret.

Mom and Dad didn't realize it at the time, but by forcing me to clean my plate, they were disturbing my innate, precious, and delicate satiety signals. They didn't know that by pushing me to override my natural ability to eat just enough and put my fork down, I would face a lifelong battle of always feeling the need to clean my plate, even if I was physically full. How could I fault them? They believed they were being responsible parents. Their intentions were so pure.

My earliest recollection of being in the clean-plate club was a dinnertime ritual whereby Mom and Dad would sneak a penny under my plate, but only if all of the food was eaten. Yes, I got paid to stuff myself.

Parents who demand their children clean their plates destroy their sense of satiety. They do this unintentionally, every day without a clue of the harmful effects they are causing. When I witness a parent insisting that a child take just one more bite, I have to resist the urge to comment.

What I really want to say is, "Please stop. Your child is a brilliant eater. Trust that, and let him tell you when he's had enough."

It's safe to say that my childhood was a pretty normal one, and my relationship with food was equally normal. I carried a healthy weight on my petite frame, balancing food with physical activity. The food wasn't portion-controlled or calorie-counted; rather, my body was its own calorie counter. A gentle grumble of my stomach signaled the need for food, while a disinterest in continuing the eating process told me it was time to stop eating. My body knew what it needed, how to get it, and what to do with it. Food was always secondary, and physical activity was called play. My body weight never crossed my mind. Even when the boys poked fun at my flat chest, my self-esteem never wavered. Sadly, it's a rare thing to be secure in one's own skin, but I was—at least for a little while.

It wasn't until my senior year in high school that I began feeling less than adequate in my own skin. I became keenly aware of my body and how it measured up to other girls my age. I was still petite, but I now looked at myself through a harsh, critical, and unloving lens. I wasn't alone; all girls my age complained about their bodies, sort of like a rite of passage into womanhood. We didn't dare call ourselves women unless we carried around a long mental list of everything we wished were different about our bodies: thinner thighs, flatter stomach, smaller nose, longer hair— the sky was the limit. Of course, we could've always chosen to love ourselves as we were, but then we'd run the risk of appearing conceited. Love *me*? Preposterous. What would they think?

I graduated from high school in the spring of 1993; it was such an exciting time for me. I couldn't wait to get out and go off to college. Looking back at some of my graduation-day photos, it was clear that I had put on weight. I wasn't overweight, but I certainly looked different. It's funny because I don't remember putting the weight on, but it was obvious that the previous months of partying with friends and filling up on alcohol and processed junk food caught up with me.

All of these bodily changes, and still I can't remember food being an issue. It remained secondary. There was one distinct difference, however; I was now conscious of my weight gain and no longer felt comfortable in my body.

College at the University of Akron was so different: no parents or rules. I thought this was something I wanted more than life itself, but I was miserable. I had no appetite whatsoever, but I knew I had to eat. A typical day of meals included a Nutrigrain bar with skim milk for breakfast, and for lunch, a small salad with ranch dressing from the pitiful iceberg-lettuce salad bar in the dining hall. Dinner consisted of a slice of pizza or cup of ramen-noodle soup.

Slowly, my body dropped the extra weight it had been holding onto for a year. I wasn't dieting or trying to lose weight; on the contrary, it was my first experience with shifting to my set point weight—the weight that the body naturally settles at when exercised regularly and fed appropriate amounts of food.

My relationship with food throughout my early college years was pretty healthy. Now, maybe I didn't choose the healthiest foods (unless pizza, diet Pepsi, and low-fat Twinkies are health foods), but food was secondary, and I felt mentally secure around it.

In the fall of 1996, I entered the field of dietetics, having a healthy relationship with food, and by graduation day in May of 2000, I had full-blown binge eating disorder. How in the world did this happen? I still find it so ironic that I went into a field that promotes health and yet was personally the unhealthiest I had ever been in my life.

"This field typically attracts women with eating disorders" was a statement confidently delivered by the head of dietetics at the University of Akron during my program orientation. I was immediately offended because at the time, I wasn't suffering from an eating disorder. Or so I thought.

The fact is, I was secretly fighting a battle with food. During that period of my life, I was focused on partying and having a good time—not unusual behavior for a woman in her early twenties. Every weekend, I frequented the Flats, a stretch of nightclubs in downtown Cleveland. Now more than ever before, my appearance was all that mattered. I became extremely conscious of my body shape, and it started to bug me. One of my best girlfriends at the time was naturally thin, and I envied her. I decided that I needed to be thinner. Why couldn't I have her body?

It's no wonder the emaciated look was the object of my desire; after all, at the time, Kate Moss was one of the highest paid supermodels. Her ninety-pound body was splattered all over the fashion magazines for young women. Thin was definitely in.

I was also on the relationship market, and the dating scene was wide open for me. I'd just ended a five-year relationship and was ready to jump into a new one—one that made me feel worth something.

Then, in the summer of 1997, it happened. There he was, standing on the dance floor in the most hopping club in the Flats—the man who would become my husband, Wayne. He was perfect in every way: striking looks, a body that most men would kill for, and a sparkling personality that lit up the room. He made me feel so very special. In fact, I remember thinking to myself, *Something has to be wrong with this guy; he's too perfect.* But that something never showed up.

We had so much fun together. But in our early days of dating, it became very clear to me that he valued thinness in a woman, which I was at the time. I was a little too thin. But of course my mind went to *I just know I can be thinner. He'll like me even more if I am.* Of course, this wasn't true, but it was a catalyst for me to achieve the body weight I just knew would make me happy.

I chose to follow a very low calorie diet. It was a starvation diet, really. Eating around a thousand calories a day and exercising for at least an hour each day, I finally reached the hundred-pound mark, which was only fifteen pounds less than the weight my body carried in a natural, nondiet state.

Don't get me wrong; nothing about this process was easy or natural. Most days, I walked around in a foggy, light-headed state. Mood swings and hunger pangs were common occurrences, and I was unhappy, to say the least. It's almost as if my body knew this wasn't good, and it simply couldn't feel right. The only thing that kept me going were the flattering comments from Wayne and other people. "Gosh, you're so thin," is poisonous rocket fuel to the brain of someone with an eating disorder. It feeds her brain with the false notion that she is loved, adored, and admired because she is thin. It perpetuates the maddening behavior of dieting and overexercising.

I must keep this up so he'll continue to like me, I thought. *If I gain any weight back, he'll notice and won't be as attracted to me. People will notice that I gained weight.*

These were the beliefs that hijacked my mind, to the point where I became obsessed with thinness. For me, the approval of others fed my very existence. I cared too damn much what other people thought. But then again, if we are really honest with ourselves, don't we all care what others think about our body, accomplishments, successes, and failures?

Just like anything in life involving stress, the more pressure that's applied, the more difficult it is for it to stay the same, and it eventually busts. I suppose nature intends for things to unfold this way. I believe it works in our favor. In my experience, that excessive pressure to stay super thin actually saved my life. I busted. I simply couldn't keep it up any longer. My body wanted so badly to be fed, and it made sure that it happened.

I can't remember the exact breaking point, but when it hit, my life was forever changed. Some people perish from the pressure. They miss the wakeup call. They ignore the cry for food, and their poor precious body gives out. It has no choice, really. I feel so blessed that my body refused to allow me to ignore it. Of course, at the time, I hated my body more and more each day because it would do everything in its power to ensure that it got fed, including participating in secret binges and thinking about food 24/7. I felt like I was going insane.

My body was only doing what it needed to live, but I didn't understand this quest for survival. I would punish it for overeating by overexercising to release the calories that it demanded and always received. It always got its way. A few times, when I was really desperate, I forced the food out with laxatives and self-induced vomiting. And then I would restrict my calories yet again to undo the damage I caused.

Essentially, I continued to starve, and when I did eat, it was fat-free or super low fat. At the time, it was a common belief that dietary fat made you fat. That's what all the popular diet books led you to believe, and of course it was supported by the US Department of Agriculture's Food Guide Pyramid, which encouraged you to eat six to eleven servings of grains every day, while minimizing fat. I took this guidance to the extreme.

Every piece of food that passed my lips had to have no more than two grams of fat inside. I paid no attention to sugar, preservatives, and other substances that were harmful to my health, only fat. Cookies, ice cream, candy, yogurt, breads, crackers, salad dressings, cakes, frostings, and peanut butter (yes, peanut butter) were all either fat-free or very low-fat. Pretzels were a staple in my diet because they were naturally fat-free. My favorite afternoon snack was twenty mini pretzel sticks and diet Pepsi. I would eat this treasured dieter's delight while sitting in my nutrition classes, learning all about proper nutrition. How's that for irony?

When Wow chips hit the grocery shelves, I just knew there was a God. They were a line of snack chips made with a fat replacement called olestra. It had all the properties of fat, including mouth feel and taste, but it went through the body undigested, so you didn't have to worry about the calories. There was one downside: A potential side effect of eating olestra was loose bowel movements. And do you think that stopped me? Hell, no. They were fat-free; they had to be good for you, I reasoned. We won't even go into how my body handled those Wow chips. I truly believed I was doing my body good.

Reflecting back during this time in my life, it's so clear to me why I craved certain nutrients, like fat. It was because my diet was devoid of them. The starve-crave-binge cycle looked something like this:

Starve myself by eating very little for breakfast, maybe a slice or two of fat-free bread with strawberry jam. Lunch was a sandwich made with the same fat-free bread, a slice of fat-free cheese, and mustard, with a piece of fruit on the side.

I would then head on over to the gym to exercise those calories off; I'd get light-headed, and as soon as I got home, the cravings would begin. Only I wasn't craving nutritious foods like blueberries, avocados, kale, and walnuts. Instead, the fat-laden, calorie-rich foods that I viewed as evil became the object of my thoughts and cravings—cake, frosting, cookies, full-fat peanut butter, and doughnuts, to name just a few.

This pressure caused an explosion of sorts within me, and the binge that followed was inevitable. I would start with one cookie, then two. Moving on over to the freezer, I'd pull out a pint of vanilla ice cream (which I didn't even really like) and then dig into any leftover pastry or cake. If there was chocolate in the house, I'd devour that too, and when I got really desperate, I would venture into our laundry room, where Mom kept her baking supplies. Tubed icing, cherry pie filling, and sprinkles became additional items on my binge menu.

Because I was feeding my body highly processed junk food, it continued to crave junk food.

I went to great lengths to conceal my daily binging habit. On our very first Easter together, Wayne presented me with a gorgeous oversized Easter basket. In the middle sat a solid milk chocolate bunny on green Easter grass, surrounded by peanut butter-filled chocolate eggs and jellybeans. And if that wasn't Willie Wonka enough, he managed to spiral a two-foot pink and yellow marshmallow rope around the handle of the basket. It was a binge-eater's dream.

The gift of that Easter basket, as deliciously special as it was, was like wrapping up a bottle of whiskey and giving it to an alcoholic for Christmas. Poor Wayne didn't know that I was fighting a ferocious battle with food and that sugar was my drug of choice.

Throughout that Easter afternoon, I disappeared up to my bedroom several times to sneak candy: a couple of peanut butter eggs here, a few handfuls of jellybeans there.

After the third trip, Wayne finally asked, "Mel, why do you keep going upstairs?"

Of course, I couldn't tell him the real reason—that I was devouring my Easter basket like a starving raccoon feasting on a post-picnic garbage can. I mean, how could I reveal to this wonderful guy that I was a junk food junkie in the middle of a completely out-of-control sugar binge? Instead, I did what any woman would do when she's trying to impress the man of her dreams: I told him my stomach was bothering me, and I had to use the bathroom. Imagine me preferring that this devastatingly handsome guy picture me on the toilet rather than eating a peanut butter egg. That's how ashamed I was.

As my life spun out of control, I became increasingly disgusted with my body, to the point where I was bordering on self-hatred. I couldn't understand these intense cravings.

I was obsessed with food; it was on my mind day and night. I even found myself overly interested in reading cookbooks.

Why couldn't I break out of this vicious cycle? Why was my mind doing this to me? It was a mystery then, but now it's very clear: my higher self was trying to keep my body alive.

I've learned that when deprived of food—which results in low blood sugar—the body will crave what it knows will raise its blood sugar. Sugar. And it will do everything in its power to break you down until you cave. Yes, the human body is brilliant, indeed. I am so very thankful that my body caved, that it won; otherwise, I wouldn't have made it. I would've perished like so many people who tragically lose their lives to eating disorders. According to the National Association of Anorexia Nervosa and Associated Disorders website, the chilling fact is that every sixty-two minutes, at least one person dies as a direct result from an eating disorder. That could've been me.

During this whirlwind of self-destruction, I found myself unable to sense fullness after a meal. I could eat for hours and hours and not feel full. I guess you could say I was numb to food. At this point, I knew I was in trouble. This lack of sensation was very foreign; it scared the living daylights out of me.

I dreamed of the day where I could go out to dinner with Wayne and eat a beautiful meal without obsession, feel comfortably full, and stop eating when I had enough. It was a craving for normalcy, to return back to days passed when food was secondary. I dreamed of this sweet day and longed to return to a place of peace with food; however, I was not at all confident that I would ever get there. In fact, I was convinced that my life from here on out would be filled with disconnect, self-abuse, and depression. A daily battle with the scale and a war against food. Food was no longer my friend; it was enemy number one, or so I thought. This ritual continued on in full force for three years.

The turning point was August 4, 2000, when Wayne and I married at the Guardian Angel Cathedral in Las Vegas, Nevada. It was a beautiful ceremony, with twenty-five of our closest friends and family members gathered to celebrate the beginning of our new life together. It should have been the most precious and blissful day of my life, but it was the furthest thing.

Don't get me wrong; marrying Wayne was the best decision I ever made. In fact, it was the only sure thing in my life at the time. But remember, up until that day, I was fighting an inner battle with myself and losing. The photos from our wedding day are proof-positive of this turmoil. They invoke feelings of sadness when I look at them because I wasn't really smiling. Sure, the photos show a half-smile, but it wasn't the kind that expressed true joy. Even when I wanted to smile big for the camera, I resisted out of fear that my face would appear puffy.

The truth is, I was sad. Sad that I was entering into this new life, with this beautiful human being, and I was out of control and completely uncertain of how I was going to manage this beast once we returned back to Ohio and moved into our new home. How would I hide it in a twelve-hundred-square-foot condominium?

As the days in Vegas wound down and we were preparing to head back home, there was one little nuisance that sat staring at me on the table in our hotel room. It was calling my name, beckoning me forth, whispering as if to say, "You think just because you're married, you can deny me? Your name may be different, but the parts are the same."

Wayne left the hotel room for a little while, and I knew this was my chance, the opportunity for one last round of mindless indulgence. I opened the box that held the top of our wedding cake; you know, the small cake that you're supposed to freeze and enjoy on your one-year anniversary? Well, our cake never saw that day.

I walked over to it and started picking at it in an all-too-familiar fashion. Guilt coursed through my veins as I inhaled a cake that I didn't even taste. After it was over, I boxed up the half-eaten evidence. When Wayne returned to the room to pack up his suitcase, he went to grab the cake box, but I immediately interfered.

"Hon, it's been sitting here, unrefrigerated for a couple of days now," I said, "and it's probably no good. Let the cleaning staff throw it away."

I certainly couldn't let him see what I'd done. What would he think? I had to preserve this perfectly controlled image, even if it killed me. As we checked out of the hotel, I had no way of knowing that the wedding cake binge would be the very last mindless splurge I'd ever experience.

We returned back to Ohio, and as we pulled up to our newly remodeled condo, life felt different. Of course, it was different in that I now lived in another city, in another home, with a man I never lived with before. It seemed like I left my old life and habits behind.

The moment I stepped over the threshold of 6830 Carriage Hill Drive, I felt transformed, like a different person. I made no conscious decision to be a different person, but all of a sudden, everything I was fighting against for the past three years dissolved. My binge eating disorder vanished as quickly as it arrived. I swear if it could talk, it would've said, "Melanie, my job here is done. You've learned everything you needed from me; goodbye."

I used to rationalize this spontaneous healing by telling people that I made a conscious decision to give up dieting. But that wasn't true. A deeper part of me knew something much bigger was responsible; I just couldn't explain it at the time.

As the years passed after my healing, little by little, I got to know myself better and developed a deeper respect for my body. No longer did I categorize food as good versus bad; instead, I made the choice to eat more wholesome foods because I knew I was worthy, and my body deserved it. I was also led to the practice of meditation to help me go within, connect with my higher self, and see myself as a woman who is healthy, healed, and in control.

I began to realize that I am so much more than what I see in the mirror. I am indeed connected to an energy so powerful, divine, expansive, and loving that it truly defies explanation. It is the source of miracles. Some may call this energy God, Universe, Source, Spirit, Nature, Tao, or Buddha. I refer to it as Divine energy.

Over an eighteen-year period, I was divinely led to discover eleven little stones, and as I turned each one over, another secret was underneath. I now call these secrets Missing Peaces. They are guidelines for living that call attention to and offer solutions for self-defeating thoughts, behaviors, and choices that keep you from fully accessing peace and well-being. When practiced, these peaces work synergistically to restore inner harmony with your food, body, and health: the real you. Think of them as tools to help you live a peaceful, healthy, and balanced life, as a human being in the real world, with temptations, food cravings, and imperfect days.

Looking back, I now realize my eating disorder was a gift, and I understand why I went through it. Partying in the Flats, meeting Wayne, dieting myself down to ninety-eight pounds, starving, binging, hitting rock bottom, dreaming of a way out, praying for a way out, in the vortex of a tornado that took my joyous life away—all so I could develop this fierce passion to help others live in peace. Had I not gone through it, I wouldn't have had the drive to turn those stones over and discover all the Missing Peaces found in this book. As a matter of fact, I wouldn't have even recognized them.

Make no mistake. These peaces are not just for those suffering from a dysfunctional relationship with their body and food. They are for anyone who has ever set out to live a healthy life but then sank back into old habits. These peaces will help you discover that your ultimate power to create better health lies within. It always has.

Path to Peace

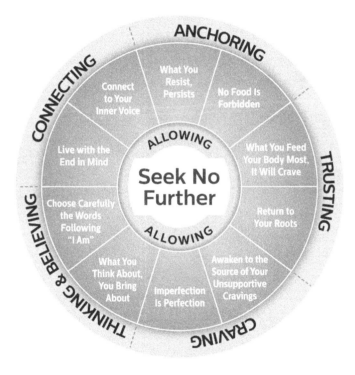

The above diagram represents what I call the Path to Peace. It contains all of the Missing Peaces you will soon experience, categorized into the following phases: Allowing, Anchoring, Trusting, Craving, Thinking and Believing, and Connecting.

In this section, I also share how, upon discovering each Missing Peace, I was able to personally restore inner harmony with my food, body, and health.

Allowing

Notice the Path to Peace doesn't look like a traditional linear path, where you start at point A, follow all the steps, and end up at your destination, which is point B. There's a very good reason for its circular shape, and it's reflected in the foundational message of Missing Peace #1: Seek No Further.

What it means is this: You are whole and complete, just as you are, and the peace you long for, that you believe is missing in your life, never went anywhere. It is never-ending and always available, when you allow it.

In this very first Missing Peace, you will learn to tune into your emotions, the barometer for whether you are connecting with Divine energy or not. To return to this good-feeling place, all you have to do is take a fully conscious breath and step into the present moment, where the peace that is your birthright forever shines.

Once you place 100 percent faith and trust in this foundational Missing Peace, you can then travel around the path to experience the ten remaining Missing Peaces. They call attention to and offer solutions for the often unconscious self-defeating thoughts, behaviors, and choices in your life that create disharmony, thereby preventing you from fully accessing peace and well-being.

Restoring Peace: This Missing Peace took me years to uncover. I was the peace all along; I just had to breathe into it and allow it. My peaceful, higher self was patiently and lovingly waiting for me to arrive, and when I finally got it, I was home.

Anchoring

The Anchoring phase of the Path to Peace includes Missing Peace #2: What You Resist, Persists and Missing Peace #3: No Food Is Forbidden. Without these understandings in place, it will be most difficult to stay on a lifelong path of healthy living. You will fight a constant battle with food and your body.

To master Anchoring, you must first learn to release all resistance to what is. This includes resistance to food and to the current state of your health and body. You must also lift the red X off of any and all foods you've ever placed it on. Freedom from food prison is the gift you receive when you give yourself permission to choose.

In this phase, you are also asked to paint a masterpiece of yourself in perfect health. This exercise opens you to the world of goodness that is not only possible for you but also inevitable, if you choose to continue your journey around the path.

Restoring Peace: Because I resisted my perfectly normal body weight by restricting food and denying my hunger, my body fought back with cravings so intense they brought me to my knees. Food won, but it was the wrong food. As I gave myself permission to choose and allowed things to just be as they were, without fighting against it, decisions involving my health and lifestyle choices became effortless, and I felt in complete control. There was a quiet knowing that all was well.

Trusting

The next stop along the path involves learning how to trust that your body knows best. This is illustrated in Missing Peace #4: What You Feed Your Body Most, It Will Crave and Missing Peace #5: Return to Your Roots.

You have so much more control over your health than you think. Did you know you were born with the magical power to crave a healthy lifestyle? The very fact that your body thrives on a steady diet of wholesome foods (what I refer to throughout the book as Earthfoods) is proof enough that it innately prefers them. This also holds true when you drink plenty of water, get adequate sleep, and engage in moderate exercise.

Your body's natural state is ease and health. It wants to be well and will do everything in its power to maintain it. However, when you make choices that don't serve you well, it knows something is wrong and, just like a cut on your finger, goes into repair mode.

The only way to crave more Earthfoods is to eat more Earthfoods, and eat them consistently. In the Trusting phase of your Path to Peace, you are guided to slowly add more of these foods to your daily meals to help you reach this state of craving.

Trusting your body means putting faith in the fact that it not only knows *what* to eat, but also *how* to eat. Babies display this instinctive behavior most brilliantly. Remember, you were once a little baby and knew exactly how much sustenance your body required to be at peace. If you are yearning to get back to that place, you must realize that your ability to sense hunger and fullness never went anywhere. Your roots are still as strong as ever. Sure, your dials may be in need of a little calibration, but rest assured, you already have within you the raw materials to make it happen.

To help you return to your roots, you are given the tools to go within and bring awareness to how much you are eating. Remember, your body knows what and how much it needs; you just have to trust it.

Restoring Peace: As I went through a gradual yet radical shift toward self-awareness, I began noticing that my body no longer wanted the foods that once held it prisoner. I also got to know myself again by connecting to and re-experiencing what hunger, satisfaction, and fullness felt like.

Craving

You are now ready to journey further around the path and learn how to navigate unsupportive cravings that often creep up without warning.

Your higher self only knows wellness. When you disturb it by overindulging in harmful substances, foods, or behaviors, it will give you a warning signal to adjust your thoughts and habits. Missing Peace #6: Awaken to the Source of Your Unsupportive Cravings will help you gain a better understanding of the origin of these cravings and offer steps you can take to stay in control.

Missing Peace #7: Imperfection Is Perfection reminds you that you are, in fact, a perfectly imperfect human being; therefore, striving for 100 percent perfection in your food choices is 100 percent unrealistic and unreasonable. Here, you are encouraged to give yourself permission to be perfectly imperfect and reframe how you approach food cravings. To guide you along, I offer a plan for successfully honoring your cravings in a healthier, more peaceful way.

Restoring Peace: I came to an understanding that certain foods nourished my body while others—no matter how pure my intentions—perpetuated addictive eating behaviors. I also learned that in order to live a truly healthy and peaceful life, free from the bonds of food prison, it was necessary for me to honor my food cravings in a healthy way, while at the same time respecting my humanness by allowing for a little bit of wiggle room.

Thinking and Believing:

In this phase of your Path to Peace, you are taken on an inner journey and asked to explore your thoughts, beliefs, and self-talk. Although you were introduced to the power of your mind in the Anchoring phase, in Missing Peace #8: What You Think about, You Bring About, you will dig even deeper to uncover any negative thoughts and make peace with those beliefs that block you from your heart's deepest desires.

If you want to know what you are thinking, examine your feelings. Really get in touch with them. How do you feel on most days? What are you getting out of life? What is the state of your health? Do they match up to your desires and wildest visions of the best you possible? If not, you will learn how to first make peace with what is and then adjust your emotions by activating a mood-booster to get you to a better feeling place. Your feelings never lie. They tell you if you're connected to who you really are in the moment or not.

Of course, you mustn't forget your spoken words, as they have tremendous power, especially when directed inward. Positive and negative words have the power to help or hinder your path to a healthier you. In Missing Peace #9: Choose Carefully the Words Following "I Am," you are given guidance on how to "change the station" from statements of negative self-talk, to those evoking better feeling thoughts.

Restoring Peace: Over time, self-love became my mission. I grew cautious of my language, refusing to use any words to describe myself that I didn't want to come to life.

I began appreciating my body for the divine temple that it is, allowing it to relax if it was tired and leading it to exercise when it was rested, because I knew it deserved both. In a sense, I became my own best friend and lover, and the only opinion of me that mattered was my own.

Connecting

Next, you experience the Connecting phase, which is making space to connect to who you really are. This is my personal favorite phase because it involves visualization and stillness, two critical pieces of my self-care routine; no matter what, they always carry me to a better place, physically and emotionally.

In Missing Peace #10: Live with the End in Mind, you are introduced to a visualization tool called the End in Mind (EIM) meditation, where you are guided to see yourself in the body of your dreams. From there, you learn how to embody that person, making the choices they would make, while believing and feeling that you already are that person. It is quite a magical experience.

In Missing Peace #11: Connect to Your Inner Voice, you learn how to tap into the voice of your higher self, the self that only knows health and peace. To do this, you must get quiet, tune in, and trust your silent, knowing observer. Meditation, which involves quieting your mind and focusing on your breath, is the most effective way to bring yourself into the present moment, where all of your power rests. When you connect to your inner voice, really settle in and listen, making healthy choices is incredibly effortless.

Restoring Peace: I started unknowingly living and making choices as if I already occupied the healthy and vibrant body of my dreams. It's almost like I couldn't even imagine my body any other way. And the beauty was, the more I lived as this person, the stronger my cravings were for good, wholesome food, exercise, and meditation.

My meditation practice has taught me to trust my feelings and emotions. When I feel good, I know I'm thinking good thoughts and moving closer to my true nature, which is peace. On the other hand, a wave of negative emotions always means a shift in my thoughts is in order. When I connect to my inner voice, making healthy choices to serve this beautiful temple I temporarily inhabit, is effortless. Meditation, connecting, breathing, living in the moment, all help to break the chains of my ego, exposing the light of my higher self.

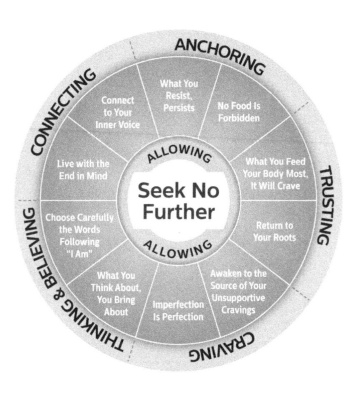

Chapter 1: Allowing

Missing Peace #1: Seek No Further

You are whole and complete just as you are, and the peace you long for, which you believe is missing in your life, never went anywhere. It is never-ending and always available, when you allow it.

In this very first Missing Peace, you will learn to tune into your emotions, the barometer for whether you are connecting with Divine energy or not. To return to this good-feeling place, all you have to do is take a fully conscious breath and step into the present moment, where the peace that is your birthright, forever shines.

Once you place 100 percent faith and trust in this foundational Missing Peace, you can then travel around the path to experience the ten remaining Missing Peaces. They call attention to and offer solutions for the often unconscious self-defeating thoughts, behaviors, and choices in your life that create disharmony, thereby preventing you from fully accessing peace and well-being.

Missing Peace #1: Seek No Further

> Peace is an attribute *in* you. You cannot find it outside.
> —*A Course in Miracles*

I used to cringe when a friend, family member, or client would come to me seeking help with their diet. Whether it was to lose weight or improve their blood sugar, I would get extremely frustrated. But not with them. I would get frustrated with myself because I couldn't help them. Sure, I prescribed a very sound meal plan and was with them every step of the way as a coach and cheerleader, but in almost every case, I noticed an eerily familiar pattern: they would follow the plan for a week or two and then fall off.

Why was it so difficult for them to stick with the plan? They were looking outside of themselves for better health: the next diet, health coach, exercise program, you name it. They failed to turn inward.

I believe the reason so many of us struggle with making lifelong healthy choices, and with our health in general, is because we have strayed off of our natural path to inner peace, or what I call home. This is a space you will only come to experience when you realize and accept that you are worthy beyond measure, when you understand that you are more than that suit of skin, bones, and blood you wear. You are the living embodiment of peace and well-being.

You were born at peace, but just like layers of dried leaves and dirt scattered about a perfectly paved pathway, your path is there; it's just been covered with years of false beliefs, forgotten power, and feelings of unworthiness.

Whatever higher power you believe in, whether you call it Divine energy, Universe, Source, God, Nature, or Spirit, *you* are directly connected to *it*. You are a piece of it, just like a fallen leaf from a majestic oak tree is indeed part of the tree. You can try to separate yourself from it, but that won't change the reality of your origin.

Because this higher power is all peaceful and exudes well-being, you too must be full of peace and health. Do you hear the simplicity of what I am suggesting to you? You are whole and complete, just as you are. You need not seek any further. The peace and well-being you long for, which you believe is missing in your life, never went anywhere. It isn't something you achieve *some* day, after you've been good and followed your diet, lost those twenty pounds, and lowered your cholesterol. It is never-ending and always available, when you allow it.

If you have been longing to reclaim the healthy and vibrant body you were meant to live in, you must catch up with this reality, stop seeking, and step into your divinity. You must allow the connection to your higher self, and with this, peace and well-being naturally shine.

So how do you know when you are connected and in a state of allowing? By paying close attention to your feelings. The way you feel is your guide to whether you are home or not. Home feels like pure, unconditional love and peace. When you are experiencing any of these emotional states, you are there:

- bliss
- clarity
- confidence
- ease
- excitement
- fearlessness
- hope
- inspiration
- joy
- love
- purpose
- passion

In contrast, negative emotions such as anger, doubt, fear, hopelessness, sadness, and worry are clear signs that you are out of alignment with your higher self and therefore disallowing peace and well-being.

Understand that positive emotions are indeed our natural states of being, but sadly, most people can't relate to them. Our tendency as human beings is to seek health, happiness, and peace as something outside of us, something we must continually strive for. We might catch ourselves saying something like, "I'll be happy and at peace when I pay off my debt [find a husband, lose these last twenty pounds, etc.]."

Chasing happiness is a futile, never-ending pursuit. Just like a dog tirelessly chasing its tail, you too will become exhausted as you continuously wait for the fulfillment of your next desire to be at peace. And sure enough, when you achieve it, you'll most certainly have another reason to withhold happiness until the next milestone is achieved.

Let us turn to Zen Master Thich Nhat Hanh for his thought-provoking solution to our endless pursuit of happiness: "There is no way to happiness; happiness is the way."

Complimenting this thought to encompass peace, Mahatma Gandhi offers us the following words: "There is no way to peace; peace is the way." Don't you see? It *starts* with peace and happiness. They are your natural emotional states. When you seek first to find peace in your heart, no matter what your current state of health, body shape, or external situation, you enter into a state of allowing and are in direct connection with who you really are. It is here you have the power to move mountains, and everything you once chased after flows to you.

I know this may sound good in theory, but what if you aren't even close to feeling happiness and peace? What if it feels like some far-off land that you will never arrive at, no matter how hard you try? What if you don't know how to feel happy?

Allowing Peace: Stepping into Presence

Make no mistake: No matter how out of control your life is, like a candle flame that never extinguishes, perfect peace is in you, always burning bright. But you don't always see it.

At any given moment, accessing your true nature, where peace and joy rest, is not only possible; it is your duty, if you wish to live in harmony with food and make wise choices to support your health. It's the only thing that will truly get you through a weak moment. And you know what? These moments aren't even weak; that's just a word we use to label something we don't have the proper tools to handle. That all changes today because I am giving you that tool right now.

Lack of presence is the only thing preventing you from claiming these gifts, yet the present moment is something available to us all. Unlocking the door into the present moment, where all of your strength and power rests, requires that you do one simple thing: take a conscious breath.

If you stop and think about it, this really makes sense, doesn't it? You can't breathe in the past or future; you can only breathe in the present moment. So the more conscious breaths you take, particularly upon making a food choice or other decision impacting your well-being, the more present you become. It is in this state where you are able to meet the larger part of you. And with this, comes the gift of peace.

I would like to take this one step further to help you really tap into the endless supply of peace that is waiting for you.

Your Light of Peace

Imagine a bright and colorful light resting inside of you, called your Light of Peace. This is the light of your higher self.

My Light of Peace is pink-lavender, a color similar to those magical sunsets that only appear every once in great while. Whenever I witness this type of glorious sunset, I enter into a deep state of serenity. Think of a color that evokes feelings of serenity deep within you; this is the color of your Light of Peace.

As you practice the art of taking a fully conscious breath in and out, picture your Light of Peace filling your entire body and then extending beyond it in every direction. Feel it as it washes over you, bathing your entire body in the warmth of its loving protection. Nothing can penetrate it or disturb you: not a bag of potato chips, a demanding boss, an overbooked schedule, or an argument with your spouse.

Negative emotions are caused by remembering a past situation or anticipating a future event, but neither one exists. When you experience any number of undesirable emotional states, like despair or doubt, it is necessary to first allow yourself to feel it for a moment and then lift the veil to discover the peace that is waiting for you. And you do this by taking a long, slow, deep breath in and out, revealing your Light of Peace. You have now entered into the present moment, where all is well. You have no worries, only peace.

Everything is possible in this state of full presence, as it is here in this light that you are connected to who you really are: your higher self.

The remaining ten Missing Peaces in this book call attention to and offer solutions for the often unconscious self-defeating thoughts, behaviors, and choices in your life that cause disharmony, thereby preventing you from fully accessing peace and well-being.

As you move through each of the phases on your Path to Peace, remember to always come back to your breath. Step into your Light of Peace, where your strength and power live. And just like a broom that with each stroke brushes the dirt away on a perfectly paved pathway, your Light of Peace will go from invisible to barely visible to bright and then blinding, with the absorption and application of each Missing Peace.

The truth is, you've held the key to inner peace and strength all along; you were just looking in all the wrong places.

Make Peace Exercise: Meet Your Higher Self

Peace and well-being are patiently waiting for your arrival today. Are you allowing it? For the next seven days, allow yourself to access these gifts on the following occasions:

1. Waking: Before getting out of bed
2. Eating: Before each meal
3. Retiring: After you climb into bed before going to sleep

To receive these gifts, step into the present moment by taking one long, slow, deep breath in and letting it out. As you take this single precious breath, see your body filling with your Light of Peace and extending beyond your body in every direction. Allow it to penetrate your every cell, molecule, and atom. Feel the difference in your emotional state (even if only slight), as you continue to breathe into your Light of Peace.

One full breath is all that is necessary, but you are welcome to take a couple more if you wish. Don't be surprised when you do because it feels really good.

Note: You may be tempted to skip one of the above moments, but stay with it. Consistency is the only way you will come to experience the full mind and body effects of tapping into this endless source of peace and well-being.

Recommended Peace of Health Shake

Chocolate Almond Cherry Shake

6 Earthfood Servings ♥ ♥ ♥ ♥ ♥ ♥
10-12 oz. unsweetened almond, cashew, coconut, or flax milk
2 tbsp. Earthfood Powder (see "Recipe" section in the back of book)
1 tbsp. raw cacao powder
1 tbsp. fresh ground almond butter
1 cup frozen organic cherries

Instructions:

Add all ingredients to a high-powered blender (such as Vitamix, Blendtec, or Ninja) in the order listed and blend until smooth.

Nutrition Facts: Calories: 385; Total Fat: 23 g; Saturated Fat: 8 g; Sodium: 160 mg; Potassium: 180 mg; Total Carbohydrates: 36 g; Dietary Fiber: 11 g; Net Carbohydrates: 25 g; Sugar: 19 g (no added sugar); Protein: 14 g

Note: Peace of Health shakes are not sweet, and that is by design. Sweetness is a trained preference, one that can be changed. The goal is to recalibrate your taste buds so that you begin to pick up the natural sweetness of the small amount of fruit in the shakes, without having to add sweetener or extra fruit. For a sweeter shake, refer to the tips offered in the "Do-It-Yourself Shakes" section at the beginning of the book.

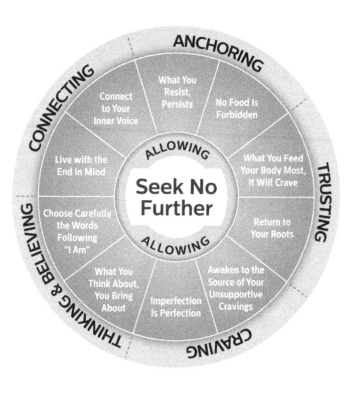

Chapter 2: Anchoring

Missing Peace #2: What You Resist, Persists
Missing Peace #3: No Food Is Forbidden

The Anchoring phase of the Path to Peace includes Missing Peace #2: What You Resist, Persists and Missing Peace #3: No Food Is Forbidden. Without these understandings in place, it will be most difficult to stay on a lifelong path of healthy living. You will fight a constant battle with food and your body.

To master Anchoring, you must first learn to release all resistance to "what is." This includes resistance to food and to the current state of your health and body. You must also lift the red X off of any and all foods you've ever placed it on. Freedom from food prison is the gift you receive when you give yourself permission to choose.

In this phase you are also asked to paint a masterpiece of you in perfect health. This exercise opens you to the world of goodness that is not only possible for you, but also inevitable if you choose to continue your journey around the Path.

Missing Peace #2: What You Resist, Persists

What you resist not only persists, but will grow in size.
—Carl Jung

When you push something away, it has a way of coming back and multiplying in strength. You may not realize this, heck, I didn't and my life would've been so much simpler had I discovered it sooner.

The best way I can describe the second Missing Peace is by comparing it to the familiar scene of a child in the grocery store checkout line. I'm sure you've witnessed a child in front of you in line, tugging at his mom's pant leg with his eye on the candy bar rack just above the conveyor belt. He tells her he wants one, but Mom quickly turns him down. Of course, that's not the answer he was hoping for, so he persists as Mom continues to deny him. In all of my grocery trips, I've yet to see this child give up and accept that he won't get the candy bar. Instead, his demands get louder; he adds a few foot-stomps and begins to throw a full-blown temper tantrum. Mom is embarrassed at the unpleasant scene as she notices everyone arching their necks to catch a glimpse of her child, who is now rolling around on the floor. Finally, she has enough and gives in, handing the candy bar to her son. He calms down, and then she realizes, he shows little interest in the treat. It was the struggle, resistance, and denial that fueled his desire for the candy bar.

In the summer of 1997, my main goal was to lose weight so that I would appear more attractive and desirable to the opposite sex. Super thin was in, so I placed myself on a very low-calorie diet.

The absence of sufficient calories forced my body into a state of physical and mental hunger that I'd never before experienced. The more I denied myself food, the stronger the drive to eat. This explains my out-of-control binging behavior at the time.

Restricting myself to a thousand calories of nutrient-poor food, such as fat-free bread, artificially sweetened yogurt, diet soda, pretzels, and multiple Sweet-n-Low packets in my already sweetened maple brown sugar oatmeal, created stronger urges to eat more than a thousand calories.

And if this wasn't damaging enough, the food I was eating to save calories ended up altering my hunger and fullness signals almost beyond repair. Research now suggests that artificial sweeteners, such as saccharin, aspartame, and sucralose, actually contribute to weight gain and elevated blood sugar.[1] So the very substance we build into our diet to help us lose weight and gain control of our health does the exact opposite.

A starvation diet, coupled with an overabundance of artificially sweetened foods, catapulted my poor body into a state of perpetual hunger and confusion. Could I have

[1] Qing Yang, "Gain Weight by 'Going Diet'? Artificial Sweeteners and the Neurobiology of Sugar Cravings." *The Yale Journal of Biology and Medicine*, June 2010.
"How Artificial Sweeteners Affect Blood Sugar and Insulin," *Healthline*, Healthline Media, February 24, 2016.

experienced success by simply changing the composition of my diet and adding more whole foods like vegetables and fruits, while increasing the calories to satisfy my hunger and cutting out the artificial sweeteners? That would've been the wise thing to do. But instead, I proceeded on this path, blaming myself for having no willpower after each defeating binge.

It turns out the very thing I was resisting—calories in the form of food—persisted in my mind, pressing until I exploded and binged. Resist sweets, the sweets persisted. It took the form of obsessive thoughts of food that I couldn't turn off. I read cookbooks and nutrition articles, not because I was interested in learning how to cook, but because of a quiet addiction that was building within. This was the obsession that eventually took my satiety signals hostage. It was as if someone disconnected the "stop eating" switch in my brain, and all of a sudden, every single piece of food that I considered to be bad became the object of my obsession. The very thing I pushed away multiplied at a reckless pace. Food had a tremendous amount of power over me. It captivated me in every sense of the word. I was consumed with it to the point where I didn't even want to get out of bed in the morning, but I knew I had to. I couldn't give up.

At the time, I didn't know how I would beat this, but something inside of me wouldn't let me give up. Days turned into months, and months turned into years, and things were getting worse. I was resisting food so much that I would binge on a daily basis. Food continued to creep into my every thought. I attempted different diets, and the results were always identical: restriction led to obsession, and obsession led to persistence of the binging behavior. For the first time in my life, I was afraid for my health and very uncertain of my future.

What you resist, persists. This is the very premise of why diets and calorie-counting fail to produce long-term results. Think about it: As human beings, we were born with a precious and precise ability to feel hunger and honor that need with just the right amount of food so the feeling disappears. We nailed this as infants. No worries at all; we figured it all out. Feel hunger, let out a cry, Mom responds by offering a bottle or her breast. We eat until we've had enough and then push the bottle or breast away. We knew what it took to satisfy our hunger. We felt it. When we had enough, there was nothing Mom could do to make us drink another drop.

Fast-forward to early childhood. If you grew up like I did, you were forced to clean your plate. No longer were we trusted to honor our brilliant, perfectly calibrated internal signals of fullness. This marks the beginning of overeating and weight gain for so many people. For me, this was the beginning of the disconnect. So as we age and gain weight, rather than tap into our once-honored innate signals of hunger and fullness, we rely on diets and calorie-counting to aid us in returning to a healthy weight. But the problem is this: No calculation in the world can tell us how much we need. We must feel it.

Unfortunately, so many of us have lost trust in ourselves and instead believe that the latest and greatest diet can save us, so we hand our power over to it. But it never really works because what you resist, persists.

I hear this all the time: "But Melanie, my last diet worked because I lost twenty pounds."

And my reply is always the same: "And where are you today? Back to the drawing board? If so, it didn't really work."

Imagine I calculate your daily calorie requirement, with the goal of helping you achieve a weight loss of one pound per week. Let's say this daily calorie level turns out to be 1200. I give you weeks of meal plans to help you stay within this range, and you plug along just fine for a few days, until you start to get hungry. Then the obsession with calories begins, which results in the subtle yet powerful loss of your ability to really connect with food. Food is no longer nourishment. It's no longer secondary. It becomes a tool to manipulate, for the purpose of shedding pounds. You find yourself choosing calorie-controlled crap foods (I like to call them CCF for short) like pretzels, crackers, and diet yogurts so you can eat more, while staying in your prescribed calorie range. Hunger builds, your mind stays focused on calories versus how your body is feeling, and you end up blowing the diet by eating a bowl of pasta or ice cream.

Sound familiar? This is what assigning power to food looks like. And when food has power, it wins every single time. No exceptions.

My philosophy on calories is that they don't matter. It's the quality of food that really counts. Popular weight-loss diets penalize the dieter when they choose a handful of walnuts over a 100-calorie pack of pretzels. After all, walnuts are rich in calories and fat, and pretzels are not; therefore, choose the pretzels, they reason. Without getting into too much of a nutrition lesson, pretzels are a pure, refined carbohydrate food (basically, they are sugar). They digest rapidly and raise your blood sugar, which subsequently drops not long after, causing a rebound hunger to occur an hour or so later. You then reach for more CCF, and the cycle repeats itself.

Now hear this: CCF is anti-weight management food. Their rapid digestion, with subsequent rise and fall of blood sugar, lays the perfect groundwork for rebound hunger, food cravings, and overeating. Take that handful of walnuts, and your body treats it much differently. Because of its fat and nutrient content, you digest it more slowly, and your blood sugar doesn't follow the same pattern as with the pretzels. It's much more controlled, which means your hunger will stay satisfied, and cravings will be absent.

The human body is in search of nutrients from food, not calories. So when you feed it loads of CCF, it begins the search for the nutrients that it knows will satisfy it. But when it can't find those nutrients, it continues to eat more, still looking.

This is precisely why, when you eat a nutrient-rich meal such as a big plate of salad greens mixed with a variety of raw veggies, along with some healthy protein like wild salmon and good fats like avocado, extra virgin olive oil, and a sprinkle of nuts or seeds, you feel completely fulfilled. You aren't likely stuffed, but what I like to call satisfied to the core. The hunger switch gets turned off because your body extracted everything it needed from that meal. This is exactly why big salads are on my dinner menu at least three nights a week. Plus, they just make me feel good.

What you resist, persists. And this goes for anything, whether it's an individual food like potato chips or grapes, or calories and food all together. The object of restriction will haunt you until it breaks you down, and you eat the entire bag. If you can get your head wrapped around this idea, you've won half of the battle.

When you resist the extra weight on your body, it will persist and even multiply. Does this mean you should be complacent and do nothing about it? Should you leave those extra fifty pounds alone and continue to eat the same foods, in the same quantities that got you there in the first place? Of course not. Am I suggesting you eat the entire bag of potato chips, because after all, it would show that you aren't resisting the chips? Now that would be just plain silly, wouldn't it?

At your core, you are whole and complete. This is the real you, your higher self, the one that knows what true wellness really is. It wants you to be healthy, vibrant, and strong. It is forgiving in nature and would never aim to make you feel ashamed for eating a few potato chips or a spoonful of ice cream. This piece of you is peace.

This is not about complacency; it's about accepting and embracing where you are right now. You don't have to love it, but you must accept and make peace with it, if you ever want to move forward. There is no other way to break free from the chains of food addiction, excess weight, or poor health than to make peace with where you're at in this moment. Release all resistance to what is.

Make Peace Exercise: Release Resistance

1. Make a list of everything you are resisting in your life. This can include your current state of health, body weight, calories for the sake of weight control, or a certain food group altogether.
2. Spend a week in quiet, peaceful acceptance of what is, and release all resistance. Journal what this process of surrendering feels like in your mind and body.

Return to Your Light of Peace

If you recall from Missing Peace #1: Seek No Further, the way to tap into this endless supply of peace and well-being is to allow yourself to be fully present for this moment. Return to your Light of Peace by taking a few long, slow, deep breaths in and out, allowing it to radiate throughout your entire body. Your light represents acceptance and love, and as you return to this place with each breath, you are resisting nothing.

Recommended Peace of Health Shake

Clean & Green Shake

6 Earthfood Servings ♥♥♥♥♥♥

10 oz. unsweetened almond, cashew, coconut, or flax milk
2 tbsp. Earthfood Powder (see "Recipe" section in the back of book)
½–1 tsp. matcha
½ tbsp. MCT oil
½ of a small avocado, peeled and seeded
2 cups fresh organic spinach
½ cup frozen mango
¼ lemon with rind

Instructions:

Add all ingredients to a high-powered blender (such as Vitamix, Blendtec, or Ninja) in the order listed and blend until smooth.

Nutrition Facts: Calories: 400; Total Fat: 31 g; Saturated Fat: 15 g; Sodium: 200 mg; Potassium: 930 mg; Total Carbohydrates: 31 g; Dietary Fiber: 15 g; Net Carbohydrates: 16 g; Sugar: 12 g (no added sugar); Protein: 14 g

Note: Peace of Health shakes are not sweet, and that is by design. Sweetness is a trained preference, one that can be changed. The goal is to recalibrate your taste buds so that you begin to pick up the natural sweetness of the small amount of fruit in the shakes, without having to add sweetener or extra fruit. For a sweeter shake, refer to the tips offered in the "Do-It-Yourself Shakes" section at the beginning of the book.

Missing Peace #3: No Food Is Forbidden

Man cannot be freed by the same injustice that enslaved it.
—Pierce Brown

If someone were to tell me twenty years ago that the key to being in the driver's seat of my food choices was to declare, and believe with everything that I am, that no food is forbidden, I would've called them insane. I now realize that without this piece, there can be no peace.

Understand that when you approach food—any food—with a mind-set of good versus evil, especially if you happen to love the evil food, you set yourself up for a dysfunctional relationship with that very food. Let's revisit the all-too-familiar weight-loss diet. Most popular diets provide you with two lists of foods: those you're allowed to eat and those you must avoid. Let's say one of the forbidden foods is Hershey's Kisses. Let's assume that up until this point, you've had a pretty healthy relationship with Hershey's Kisses, eating maybe one or two every day with no guilt. But once that Hershey's Kiss is placed on the forbidden list, it takes on a different form. No longer is it a harmless Hershey's Kiss; it now takes the identity of your warden, holding your thoughts prisoner. It trains you to think and obsess about it night and day, even showing up in your dreams.

It's an unnatural feeling of powerlessness, and you can't quite figure out why. Eventually, you break down and buy a bag of Kisses—because food always wins under these conditions—and soon, you're sitting in the middle of a pile of foil wrappers, wondering what went wrong. It was like an out-of-body experience. That once-peaceful relationship you had with the Hershey's Kiss has turned into an all-out dysfunctional and abusive one.

There is something you must understand: The Hershey's Kiss did nothing wrong; it was just being a Kiss. You were the one who changed. You went from being an independent thinker to single-handedly giving power and permission to food, permission to rule your thoughts, beliefs, and feelings.

The question now becomes, how do you return to that peaceful state where you once viewed a Hershey's Kiss as just a Kiss, a lump of chocolaty goodness, instead of a tyrant? The key is, you must view the Kiss, and every other food on the face of the planet, as allowed. You must lift the proverbial red X off all foods you've ever placed it on, including potato chips, chocolate, ice cream, cheeseburgers, and, yes, Kisses. This is the only way to unlock your prison door, and the amazing thing is, you've held the key all along.

What are the signs that you've finally broken free from the chains of food? You can refuse dessert at your favorite restaurant and not feel like a caged animal that really wants the chocolate mousse cake, but knows she shouldn't. You just really didn't want it. You can go for ice cream, order a scoop of your favorite flavor, and savor every last bite without an ounce of guilt or regret. You can walk past a bowl of Hershey's Kisses, not take one, and not want one. And if you *do* want one, you are in complete control and can eat just one or two and feel mentally satisfied. Could you eat another one? Of course, but because you took away its sex appeal, you extinguished the fire of desire for that very food.

Are you making the connection yet of how close this Missing Peace is to the previous one: What You Resist, Persists? If you resist the Kiss because some diet placed it on the forbidden list, it will persist in your thoughts and dominate your life. When you take the red X off of the Kiss and declare (and believe in your gut), "I can have this Kiss if I want it," you, my friend, have taken your power back. And what a sweet day that will be.

I don't want you to misunderstand me here. I'm not suggesting that you go to the grocery store and fill up your cart with any and all foods you've ever forbidden yourself from eating: doughnuts, cupcakes, cookies, frozen pizza, and so on. But what I do want to make clear to you is that it is your right to do so, if you choose. None of these foods are off-limits to you.

Try this little experiment the next time you go grocery shopping: take your cart down all of the aisles and departments housing your favorite, previously off-limit foods, and declare them allowed. For example, I push my cart through the bakery, past the doughnut, cookie, cake, and brownie cases, and mentally announce the following: *I can totally have that doughnut if I really want it. I can so fill my cart up with brownies and white chocolate macadamia nut cookies if I really wanted them. I have the freedom to put into my cart anything I choose.* This simple act has a way of unraveling the chains and unlocking the door to your food prison cell, allowing you the freedom that is your birthright. Now, you can breathe.

The crucial key to this experiment is that you must believe, deep down in your soul, that you can have these foods if you really want them. The question is, do you really want them now that you know you can have them? I can almost hear you: *Well, of course I want it, Melanie. I mean, who wouldn't choose a warm glazed doughnut over an apple or a brownie over a banana?* Again, it is your choice; there's nothing and no one stopping you. But first, I invite you to consider your vision of perfect health.

If you could create a body in perfect health, what would that look and feel like? Would you have any aches and pains? How would your blood pressure look? What about the shape of your body; would you create a shape that is layered in fat or toned and flexible? My guess is that you would create a masterpiece of health. So it stands to reason that a body in perfect health would be fueled and sustained by healthy, natural foods from the earth, like vegetables, fruits, nuts, and seeds, rather than human-made food shoved into boxes and cans.

It is your choice at the end of the day, and if you consciously choose to eat foods that, over time, can damage your health, you are the one who will have to face the consequences. Remember, you are accountable to one and only one person: yourself. So you will have to answer to yourself when making choices that are incompatible with your higher self.

When you make choices that are out of alignment with the desires of your higher self, you feel disconnected and weak. Whereas when you make choices that serve and honor the *real* you, it feels like clarity, joy, energy, and pure bliss—like all is right in the world, and nothing is missing.

The beauty of achieving that perfect health you've painted in your mind is, you don't have to be a perfect eater to get there. All it takes is one small change to get you on the path. You can build momentum from there.

Many people have a legitimate concern that you too may share: What if you don't like the taste of spinach, broccoli, quinoa, or blueberries? What if even the thought of drinking a glass of water is enough to make you want to gag? What if your taste buds are so used to cheeseburgers, potato chips, and peanut butter cups that you think there's no hope for you ever getting to a place in your life where you are eating wholesome, nutritious foods on a daily basis, much less enjoying them? This brings me to the next Missing Peace: What You Feed Your Body Most, It Will Crave.

Make Peace Exercise: Allow All Food

1. The next time you go grocery shopping, take your cart down all of the aisles and departments housing your favorite, previously off-limit foods and declare them allowed. How did this make you feel?

2. Build the masterpiece that is you. If you could create a body in perfect health, what would that body look and feel like? It's very important that you

get specific here and let your imagination go wild. Pretend you are painting a piece of art to be hung in an art museum, next to Picasso and Monet.

a. What does your body look like?
b. What does your body feel like (toned, smooth, energetic, flexible, strong)?
c. What is the state of your health (blood pressure, cholesterol, blood sugar, heart, lungs, kidneys, liver, etc.)?

Return to Your Light of Peace

As you take a few conscious breaths and connect with your Light of Peace, see the masterpiece that is you. Breathe into the desires of your higher self. When faced with a decision about what to eat, breathe into your Light of Peace and ask yourself, Will eating this food brighten or dull my light? Will it energize or weaken me? Is this food worthy of going into my body at this moment?

Recommended Peace of Health Shake

Ginger Pear Shake

7 Earthfood Servings ♥♥♥♥♥♥♥

10 oz. unsweetened almond, cashew, coconut, or flax milk
2 tbsp. Earthfood Powder

1 tbsp. fresh ginger

½ tsp. cinnamon

1 tbsp. coconut butter

½ cup carrots

1 cup fresh sliced organic pears (with skin on)

Instructions:

Add all ingredients to a high-powered blender (such as Vitamix, Blendtec, or Ninja) in the order listed and blend until smooth.

Nutrition Facts: Calories: 375; Total Fat: 23 g; Saturated Fat: 15 g; Sodium: 200 mg; Potassium: 490 mg; Total Carbohydrates: 38 g; Dietary Fiber: 14 g; Net Carbohydrates: 24 g; Sugar: 20 g (no added sugar); Protein: 10 g

Note: Peace of Health shakes are not sweet, and that is by design. Sweetness is a trained preference, one that can be changed. The goal is to recalibrate your taste buds so that you begin to pick up the natural sweetness of the small amount of fruit in the shakes, without having to add sweetener or extra fruit. For a sweeter shake, refer to the tips offered in the "Do-It-Yourself Shakes" section at the beginning of the book.

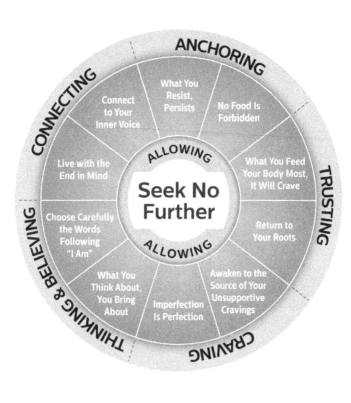

Chapter 3: Trusting

Missing Peace #4: What You Feed Your Body Most, It Will Crave

Missing Peace #5: Return to Your Roots

The next stop along the path involves learning how to trust that your body knows best. This is illustrated in Missing Peace #4: What You Feed Your Body Most, It Will Crave, and Missing Peace #5: Return to Your Roots.

You have so much more control over your health than you think. Did you know you were born with the magical power to crave a healthy lifestyle? The very fact that your body thrives on a steady diet of wholesome foods (what I refer to throughout the book as Earthfoods) is proof enough that it innately prefers them. This also holds true when you drink plenty of water, get adequate sleep, and engage in moderate exercise.

Trusting your body means not only putting faith in the fact that it knows *what* to eat, but also *how* to eat. To help you return to your roots, you are given the tools to go within and bring awareness to how much you are eating. Your body knows what and how much it needs; you just have to trust it.

Missing Peace #4: What You Feed Your Body Most, It Will Crave

> Habit is habit, and not to be flung out of the window
> by any man, but coaxed downstairs one step at a time.
> —Mark Twain

This is one of the most empowering Missing Peaces I can share with you.

Do you realize how amazing your body is? It has the ability to adapt to any number of dietary combinations forced upon it. It has to; after all, your survival depends on it.

I want you to take a moment to think about all the foods you crave on a daily basis. These are the must-have foods in your life. When I ask this question of audience members, I usually get answers like chocolate, potato chips, French fries, and pizza. But there's always that one person who shouts out, "Salad."

So what gives? Are these salad-cravers freaks of nature? Not at all.

No matter what your food cravings, I want you to know that you orchestrated every last one of them. You are responsible for the foods your body is demanding at this moment. In reality, the individual who craves chocolate and the one who craves salad have both trained their bodies to prefer these foods. It's not about willpower; it's a matter of how frequently you put the food into your body and the physical cravings that emerge over time.

Your taste buds become trained, by you, to crave the very foods you are placing upon them. They know no better. Understand, however, that we have one strike against us from day one: We were born with a preference for sweet. It's hardwired in our brain. We didn't come out of the womb craving brussels sprouts and broccoli; it's something we have to train ourselves to crave.

This is wonderful news because it means no matter how horrible your diet is right now, you can totally transform it (and your body) by doing one simple thing: start feeding it wholesome food. That's it.

I'm not telling you to take anything out; I'm asking you to add, and add consistently. This means that if you choose to add a serving of vegetables to your diet, you must do it every single day in order to strengthen your craving for vegetables.

Cementing a craving in place can take anywhere from two weeks to two months, so whatever you do, don't give up on it. I promise, your body will respond favorably, for it is the law.

My breakfast for the past ten years has been a wholesome Peace of Health shake. The recipe changes from time to time; however, my current addiction is one chock-full of fresh avocado, kale, lemon (peel and all), ginger, turmeric root, frozen blueberries, and cauliflower (yes, cauliflower), and a homemade protein powder made of ground hemp, flax, and pumpkin seeds and naturally sweetened with cinnamon and raw cacao powder. When I don't have my smoothie due to travelling or when I replace it with an omelet on Sunday morning, I really miss it. My body literally craves it.

Earthfoods: Nutrient-Rich Foods from the Earth

What exactly are these Earthfoods I've been building up? They are the foods your body was designed to eat and truly longs for. They are powerful beyond measure and can heal your body at a cellular level.

Earthfoods include whole, plant-based, nutrient-rich foods from the earth such as vegetables, fruits, nuts, seeds, avocados, legumes, herbs, spices, cacao, and green tea. A complete list of Earthfoods can be found in the appendix for your reference.

The payoff of eating an Earthfood-rich diet is a body that is satiated to the core. These foods won't cause you to raid the refrigerator looking for more food an hour after you've eaten them (think potato chips and chocolate chip cookies). Moreover, you aren't likely to feel the need to overeat them because they are so nourishing. They give you energy, help your brain function at optimal levels, and provide a sense of clarity.

You feel so good on a steady diet of these foods that after a while, you begin to notice two things: First, you can't believe how crappy you were feeling before. Think about it; if you've always felt a certain way, you have no way of knowing how bad you really feel because you have nothing to compare it to. Or maybe it was such a gradual shift toward feeling crummy that you didn't even notice the subtle differences over the years. Maybe you just blamed it on getting old.

The second thing you'll notice after eating more Earthfoods is, when you stray off course, and processed foods begin to sneak back into your life, your body doesn't like it. It responds by manifesting little aches and pains, stomach discomfort, skin problems, digestive issues, and even brain fog.

I'm always delighted when someone tells me that they ate a few chicken wings or pizza at a party and suffered a stomachache or some other minor side effect. It's not because I'm happy they are in pain; rather, I am elated because I know these are signs that they've made a shift in their body. They've trained their body to crave the good stuff and reject the rest.

Since this isn't a diet book, I'm not going to offer you meal plans or strict rules to follow. Instead, I'll share guidelines and suggestions to help you easily implement more Earthfoods into your dietary routine to help your body crave these foods.

Consistency is critical to your success, so please be diligent about adding more Earthfoods to your daily diet. If you begin by eating a serving of two of Earthfoods at breakfast, continue doing so. They don't have to be the same ones; in fact, I encourage you to mix it up and incorporate new foods at every opportunity. Just make sure to stick to that pattern of consistency.

A serving of Earthfood is any one of the following:

- 1 cup of fresh or frozen vegetables
- 2 cups of leafy greens: kale, collard greens, spinach, Romaine lettuce, arugula, mustard greens, Swiss chard, microgreens, and so on
- ½ cup of fruit
- ½ cup cooked legumes: beans, peas, lentils
- ¼ cup nuts and seeds: walnuts, almonds, pecans, pistachios, pumpkin seeds, sunflower seeds, and so on
- 1 tbsp. of chia seeds, flaxseed, hemp seeds, sesame seeds
- 1 tbsp. of nut or seed butter: almond, cashew, peanut, macadamia nut, sunflower, and so on
- ½ of a small avocado
- 1 tbsp. of unrefined coconut oil
- 1 tbsp. fresh or 1 tsp. dried herbs and spices

To illustrate what this looks like in an actual meal, let's take a look at Melanie's Go-To Power Shake. This shake contains eight servings of Earthfoods. Unless noted, each of the following shake ingredients represent one Earthfood serving:

- 1 tsp. maca powder
- 2 tbsp. Earthfood Powder (two Earthfood servings)
- 1 tbsp. fresh ginger
- 1 tbsp. fresh turmeric
- ½ of a small avocado
- 2 cups fresh organic kale
- ½ cup frozen wild blueberries

I have full confidence that you will love the way you look and feel so much that adding more Earthfoods will become a natural progression. The more you eat them, the more you'll crave them.

Why No Food Rules?

There are two reasons why I refuse to lay down a bunch of rules about avoiding certain foods. First, I understand human nature. Humans thrive on the ability to choose, and if I take that away from you, it will only fuel your fire of desire to eat the not-so-healthy stuff. Remember the example I shared in an earlier Missing Peace, about the persistent child in the grocery store checkout line who desires a candy bar that his mom refuses to purchase? Instead, I will share the foods that will rock your health and those that rob you of it, and then let you decide.

Remember that what you eat, you crave. So if you want to begin craving healing foods, all you have to do is eat them, and do so consistently. I trust you will do what is best for you.

The second reason I am against rigid rules is because I am a realist. We live in the real world, and there will be times when the not-so-healthy foods wind up on our plate. The last thing I want you to do is beat yourself up over eating these foods. Instead, if and when you eat them, do so consciously and intentionally. Be fully aware that you are feeding your body foods that can potentially rob you of good health, if you eat too much. Just the act of being conscious of what you are eating can be enough to help you shift back toward your Earthfood-rich diet. No harm done.

Do you see how much more peaceful this approach is? For example, one of the foods I adore is cheese. I love how it tastes with a glass of dry red wine, accompanied by olives, marcona almonds, and some fresh berries. Is cheese an Earthfood? I wish. I know that eating cheese isn't particularly good for my health, but I enjoy it in moderation: an ounce or so about five days a week. Even though it's not a health-rocking Earthfood, I find a way to include it because it feeds my soul. I eat it without guilt, savoring every last bite, and then make sure the rest of my food is clean and nutrient-rich the remainder of the day. See how this works? So if I'm planning on eating cheese in the evening, I fill my breakfast, lunch, and any snacks with Earthfoods, not cheese. This is how I've been able to stay on track and binge-free all these years. It's also how I am able to stand proud and pronounce my craving for brussels sprouts, broccoli, and blueberries.

How to Make a PeaceMeal

Planning healthy meals is key to creating healthy food cravings. I only have one rule when it comes to meal planning, and I think you're really going to like it: Simply build your meals to include a minimum of three servings of Earthfoods. Three is the magic number to turn any meal into what I call a PeaceMeal.

I find that when too many rules are applied to meal planning, it just complicates what should otherwise be a fun, nurturing experience. Surely anyone can choose three Earthfoods to make a meal. Take a look at these sample meal plans, and see how easy it is. The number beside each food indicates the number of servings of Earthfoods it provides.

PeaceMeal Breakfast

Three-egg omelet made with

- 1 cup of sautéed vegetables: **1**
- 1 tbsp. fresh basil: **1**
- Served with ½ cup fresh blackberries: **1**

Coconut flour pancakes made with

- ¼ cup chopped walnuts: **1**
- 1 tsp. cinnamon: **1**
- ½ cup diced apple: **1**

Peace of Health Tropical Turmeric Shake made with

- 1 tbsp. fresh turmeric: **1**
- 1 tbsp. fresh ginger: **1**
- 2 cups fresh kale: **1**

PeaceMeal Lunch

Oversized salad made with

- 4 cups of fresh spinach and arugula: **2**
- ¼ cup unsalted pumpkin seeds: **1**

Chicken salad with

- 1 cup of chopped celery and red onion: **1**
- ½ cup cooked lentils: **1**
- 1 tbsp. fresh parsley: **1**

Egg salad on a bed of greens with

- ½ of a small avocado, mashed (used instead of mayonnaise): **1**
- 1 cup red pepper strips and baby carrots: **1**
- 1 small organic apple: **1**

PeaceMeal Dinner

Salmon fillet with

- Wild rice pilaf made with ¼ cup walnuts: **1**
- 2 cups roasted brussels sprouts: **2**

Zucchini noodle spaghetti made with

- 2 cups of spiralized zucchini: **2**
- Topped with 1 cup of broccoli: **1**

Oven-roasted organic chicken and vegetables made with

- 2 cups of veggies (bell peppers, onion, mushrooms, eggplant, cauliflower): **2**
- 1 tbsp. fresh spices: **1**

What about Protein and Fat?

To help balance your blood sugar and keep you satisfied, this is my recommendation:

1. Fill half of your plate with mostly nonstarchy vegetables, such as brussels sprouts, broccoli, greens, and cauliflower.
2. Reserve a quarter for some high-quality protein, like free-range eggs, sustainably caught wild salmon, organic free-range chicken or turkey, or organic grass-fed beef. Meatless sources of protein include legumes, nuts, seeds, tempeh, and quinoa.
3. Add some healthy fats, such as extra virgin olive oil, to dress your salad or the raw pumpkin seeds you sprinkle over your roasted brussels sprouts.

Drink Water, Crave Water

Water makes up over 50 percent of your body and about 80 percent of your brain. So whether you like the taste or not, the fact is, you can't live without it.

Many calculations exist for determining how much water you should be drinking on a daily basis. I have found, however, that the most reliable way to test hydration status is to simply look at the color of your urine. If it's pale yellow and almost clear, you are pretty well hydrated. On the other hand, if your urine is the color of apple juice or beer, this is a sure sign that you are dehydrated and need to drink more water.

Understand that your water requirements fluctuate based on several conditions. Hot weather, illness, and exercise all demand that you drink more water. Just take a quick peek at your urine color and let that be your guide.

If you aren't crazy about the taste of water, you can most certainly change this. Just like with food, when you drink water as your main beverage, your body will crave water, and no other beverage will do the trick—not juice, soda, artificially flavored water, iced tea, or sports drinks.

I used to drink very little water; instead, diet soda was my go-to thirst quencher. It's been almost twenty years since I've kicked these artificially sweetened drinks to the curb, and if I happened to take a sip of one today by accident, my taste buds get an immediate shock, and I have to drink a cup of water to cleanse my palate. Today, these drinks are downright offensive to my body. In Missing Peace #6: Awaken to the Source of Your Unsupportive Cravings, you'll learn why it's so important to eliminate artificial sweeteners from your life.

To help your body get to this water-craving state, start by squeezing a slice of lemon, lime, or orange into your water. To change things up a bit, I like to make my own fruit-infused water.

To try this for yourself, simply toss your choice of thoroughly washed and sliced fruit into a tall glass pitcher. Watermelon, cantaloupe, strawberries, pineapple, oranges, kiwi, grapefruit, apples, raspberries, blueberries, and blackberries are all wonderful. Next, fill the pitcher with water and allow to sit in the refrigerator for at least two hours. When you're ready for a drink, simply pour from the strainer side of the lid so that the fruit remains in the pitcher. For some really unique flavor combinations, try adding fresh herbs like lavender, basil, sage, lemongrass, mint, cilantro, or rosemary. If you want to get the most flavor from your fruit-infused water, consider using a muddler (or the handle of a wooden spoon) to mash the fruit and herbs a bit before you add the water.

The bottom line is this: Water is the best way to hydrate that beautiful body of yours. But to crave it, you must drink it, and drink it often.

A Note of Caution about Fruit

I'm a big fan of it, but in small amounts. It is totally healthy to include a bit a fruit in your daily diet, but I would recommend capping it at one to two servings. A serving is about a half-cup, or half of a medium to large piece of fruit (a smaller portion compared to what you may be used to).

Yes, fruit is healthy and filled with fiber and valuable vitamins, minerals, and antioxidants, but your body still breaks them down into sugar. Of course, the extra fiber that is found in fruit is a blessing because it serves to lessen the rise in blood sugar as compared to table sugar, but at the end of the day, your body treats them the same.

Chronic Inflammation: The Driver behind Diabetes, Cancer, and Heart Disease

A regular diet of low-quality food not only stimulates cravings for these very foods but also results in chronic inflammation, which underlies most major diseases, like diabetes, cancer, and heart disease.

There are two types of inflammation: acute and chronic. Typically, when we think of something in our body being inflamed, images of a cut finger or skinned knee appear in our mind. When we experience an injury like this, there's no doubt that the affected area is inflamed. It shows telltale signs of bleeding, redness, and pain. Our body then does exactly what it was designed to do: White blood cells rush to the injury site, where they perform the role of cleaning up the wound. Our blood clots, and eventually, a scab forms to seal the abrasion to keep harmful microorganisms at bay. The injury and resulting inflammation just described is called acute inflammation, a necessary process that our body must get right; otherwise, we would die.

I sometimes just sit in amazement at the wonder of the human body. It knows exactly what to do to heal and protect itself. Its only role is to keep us alive, at any cost. In January of 2015, I personally experienced the miraculous healing abilities of the human body when I set out to take a walk on an icy morning. About five minutes into my walk, I hit a patch of black ice, slipped backward, and landed directly on my butt. Hoping to break my fall and protect my head, I instinctively shot my left arm out behind me, resulting in a fractured wrist. This is an example of acute inflammation.

Let's now talk about chronic inflammation. This type of inflammation is much more worrisome because, unlike acute inflammation, where you can see and feel it, the chronic type lies silent in the body, so you really have no idea it's even happening.

Similar to acute inflammation, chronic inflammation is triggered when something is off-balance in the body, which then activates inflammatory markers to heal the perceived injury. A notable difference between the two, however, is that acute inflammation responds because of a physical injury, while chronic is attempting to heal something that isn't physically broken. It's like a warning signal that flares up in response to your lifestyle habits, only the warning signal is silent. And because, unlike a broken wrist, we can't see or feel the early stages of these diseases, chances are you will carry on as if nothing is off-balance. Then one afternoon, you walk into your doctor's office for your annual checkup, and she breaks the news that you have prediabetes.

Inflammation is fueled when you skimp on sleep and eat a diet rich in heavily processed foods, like fast food, frozen meals, and sweets, and deficient in Earthfoods. It thrives in the bodies of people who use tobacco or avoid physical exercise.

Let me be very clear on this: most chronic inflammation is caused by our choices and habits, those we repeat on a daily basis.

The very fact that your body thrives on Earthfoods, and you begin to crave them when eaten consistently, is proof positive enough that your body prefers them. When you make choices over time that do not serve you, your body knows something is wrong and, just like a cut on your finger, goes into repair mode. Its natural state is ease and wellness. It wants to be well and will do everything in its power to maintain it. When you ignore the eventual signs of disease (high blood sugar, high cholesterol), it has no choice but to be in dis-ease. This is good news because it means you have so much more control over your health than you think.

Peace for Diabetes

You've probably noticed what seems to be an epidemic of diabetes in the United States. What used to be referred to as adult-onset diabetes is now called type 2 diabetes, since it doesn't only affect adults. Young children and teens are now being diagnosed with type 2 diabetes at alarming rates, and it isn't due to genetic factors, either. The rise in processed foods and simple sugars, coupled with a sedentary lifestyle, creates the perfect storm for a diabetes diagnosis.

Intentionally building your meals around fibrous Earthfoods, with just a touch of fruit, allows your body to manage the amount of sugar it must process. And because all carbohydrate-containing foods break down into sugar, we want to be mindful that we don't feed it an overabundance of high-carbohydrate foods in one sitting. For me, this works out to be around six to seven cups of mostly nonstarchy vegetables per day and one cup of fruit. I especially like berries because they are low glycemic and house an abundance of antioxidants.

The glycemic index is a measure given to a carbohydrate-based food that reflects its effect on your blood sugar. The higher the glycemic index, the more sharply it raises your blood sugar. The glycemic index is affected by several factors, including how ripe a fruit or vegetable is when you eat it (more ripe = higher glycemic index), how processed the food is (more processed/refined/added sugars = higher glycemic index), and how long it is cooked (longer cooking time = higher glycemic index).

Low glycemic carbohydrate-based Earthfoods include

- nonstarchy vegetables,
- leafy greens,
- avocados,
- berries,
- apples,
- pears,
- grapefruit,
- beans,
- lentils,
- nuts, and
- seeds.

The amount of fiber in food also helps to slow the release of sugar in the blood. This is why I suggest you load up on Earthfoods—they are naturally high in fiber.

In addition, as noted above, when eaten with protein and fat-rich foods, carbohydrate foods will digest more slowly, therefore reducing the impact on your blood sugar. For example, eating a bowl of pasta with marinara sauce will spike your blood sugar within an hour after it's eaten. If you reduce the amount of pasta in that bowl and top it off with 3–4 oz. of organic, free-range chicken, or a couple of grass-fed beef meatballs, and serve it alongside a generous leafy green salad drizzled with extra-virgin olive oil and sprinkled with raw walnuts, you will have much better control over your blood sugar.

If you have been diagnosed with prediabetes or type 2 diabetes, my recommendation is to follow the guidelines I offered earlier: a minimum of three Earthfood servings per meal, including lots of nonstarchy vegetables (two servings of fruit per day or less), and then adding a few ounces of healthy protein and a moderate amount of fat. Don't forget to cook with plenty of fresh herbs and spices too.

Although those with type 1 diabetes can benefit greatly from the meal-planning guidelines outlined above, it is best to check with your health care provider first, as insulin and other medications may need to be adjusted.

The simplicity of this meal-planning method makes it easy to follow long-term. Gone are the days of counting calories and carbohydrates.

Also, I must mention that whatever you do, be sure to enjoy your food. Really taste and savor every bite. Food is meant to be enjoyed, so let's not forget that.

Peace for Heart Disease and Cancer

Now that we covered diabetes, what about heart disease and cancer? How should you be eating to prevent these two major diseases that claim the lives of thousands upon thousands of people each year?

The answer is simple: You needn't change a thing. At the end of the day, a diet rich in Earthfoods will help create health in your body, which means it lessens the risk for not only diabetes, but also heart disease and cancer.

The Earthfood-rich environment you create in that beautiful body of yours is a threatening atmosphere for disease. What I'm saying is this: Eat more Earthfoods, crave more Earthfoods. Crave more Earthfoods, create more health, and discourage inflammatory diseases from taking up residence in your body.

Rather than wait for a diagnosis, why not get in the driver's seat of your health and take small steps to create health in your body?

"I Want to, but It's Just Too Difficult"

One of the most common beliefs about improving our health is that it's too difficult. Too difficult to eat healthy; after all, we are so busy nowadays, most people barely have enough time to brush their teeth, let alone prepare healthy meals. Or do they?

Consider this: What if every excuse you've been feeding yourself about how difficult life is, is just a big fat lie? What if it's easy, and we've just convinced ourselves it's tough? It really is a matter of perspective. What were you raised to believe? What do your friends say and believe about living a healthy life? "No pain, no gain"? Or how about "It takes too much effort to eat healthy," or "I don't have time to exercise"?

If you tell yourself something long enough, you really do start to believe it. It becomes your reality. But why not choose a different reality?

Wayne Dyer offered this thought in his book *Excuses Begone!:*[2]

> You have absolutely no incontrovertible evidence that what you'd like to change is actually going to be challenging. It's just as likely to be easy for you to change your thinking as it is to be hard.

---

[2] Wayne W. Dyer, *Excuses Begone!: How to Change Lifelong, Self-Defeating Thinking Habits.*

He goes on to say,

> The belief that [your habits are] going to be hard to change is only a belief! Making something difficult in your mind before you even undertake the effort is an excuse. As an ancient Taoist master once concluded: Nothing in the world is difficult for those who set their mind to it.

Still, you may not believe it's easy to eat more vegetables when they taste bland or even offensive. But this is where you must trust and have faith in this Missing Peace; what you feed your body most, it will crave.

You only have to move the needle just a little bit in the direction of self-care, and your body will demand more. I'm not talking about moving mountains here; just little piles of dirt.

I challenge you to consider the idea that to stay the same is more difficult than making a single change that can create health and harmony in your body.

Make Peace Exercise: Eat Earthfoods, Crave Earthfoods

1. Write down all of the foods you crave on a daily basis.
2. Rather than forbid yourself of any food you currently crave, name at least ten Earthfoods you would like to crave, and begin adding them to your meals (see

appendix for a complete list of Earthfoods). This works out to a minimum of three Earthfoods per meal. For example, ginger, carrots, and pears could easily be incorporated into your morning Peace of Health shake.

3. Make a promise to yourself right now that you will begin feeding that beautiful body of yours at least three Earthfoods at each meal, and repeat until you begin to crave it or miss it when you don't have it.

Return to Your Light of Peace

Once again, take a long, slow, deep breath in, and let it out. Repeat this cycle of conscious breathing until you feel your colorful Light of Peace shining bright within you. In this place, it is very clear that your body wants to be well. Your higher self desires nourishing, life-sustaining foods that will bring it energy.

As you sit down to enjoy a PeaceMeal, pause to take another breath. Return to your Light of Peace, where you can be fully present with the food that is before you. With every bite of Earthfood you take, see the flames of chronic inflammation slowly extinguish. Feel your body absorb the nutrients, and observe your cells as they begin to crave these foods.

Recommended Peace of Health Shake

Tropical Turmeric Shake

7 Earthfood Servings ♥ ♥ ♥ ♥ ♥ ♥ ♥

12 oz. unsweetened coconut milk
2 tbsp. Earthfood Powder
¼ lime, with rind
1 tbsp. fresh turmeric
1 tbsp. fresh ginger
¼ of a small avocado, peeled and seeded
½ tbsp. MCT oil
2 cups fresh organic spinach or kale
¼ cup frozen pineapple
¼ frozen banana or ¼ cup frozen mango
Organic, unsweetened coconut flakes (sprinkled on top of prepared smoothie)

Instructions:

Add all ingredients to a high-powered blender (such as Vitamix, Blendtec, or Ninja) in the order listed and blend until smooth.

Nutrition Facts: Calories: 400; Total Fat: 30 g; Saturated Fat: 15 g; Sodium: 190 mg; Potassium: 540 mg; Total Carbohydrates: 34 g; Dietary Fiber: 11 g; Net Carbohydrates: 23 g; Sugar: 10 g (no added sugar); Protein: 13 g

Melanie M. Jatsek, RD, LD

Note: Peace of Health shakes are not sweet, and that is by design. Sweetness is a trained preference, one that can be changed. The goal is to recalibrate your taste buds so that you begin to pick up the natural sweetness of the small amount of fruit in the shakes, without having to add sweetener or extra fruit. For a sweeter shake, refer to the tips offered in the "Do-It-Yourself Shakes" section at the beginning of the book.

Missing Peace #5: Return to Your Roots

> Deep in their roots, all flowers keep the light.
> —Theodore Roethke

I love watching babies. It fascinates me how they explore all areas of life with such energetic wonder. I especially enjoy observing them at mealtime and all of the little moments leading up to it.

First, they fuss a little bit, bringing their hand up to their mouth, smacking their lips while letting out little sucking noises. Still, they are at peace; just a little hunger, no big deal. Of course, if that hunger is not satisfied soon, panic begins to set in, and the crying begins. At this moment, they are temporarily uncomfortable, but the feeling dissipates the moment Mom comes rushing to the scene with breast or bottle. As baby's tummy fills up, she relaxes back into her peaceful state, and you can see that all is right again in her little world.

My favorite part of the infant feeding process is watching the baby refuse the rest of the bottle after she has had enough. How does she do it? How does she know that a 3-oz. bottle is enough? Not 2 or 3.5 oz., but 3. Moreover, why doesn't she feel the need to clean her plate?

I sometimes sit in amusement as I observe a well-meaning mom or dad trying with all of their might to get baby to empty the bottle. They do everything short of standing on their head, but still, she refuses to drink another drop; 3 oz. is all her little body requires to return to a state of peace.

Babies are the most brilliant eaters of all. They really have it figured out. Don't you see? You were once that little baby and knew exactly what your body needed to be at peace. But if you grew up like me, you were raised and encouraged (and, in my case, even paid) to clean your plate, so you slowly unlearned your brilliance.

If you are yearning to get back to that place, you must realize that your ability to sense hunger and fullness never went anywhere. Your roots are still as strong as ever. Sure, your dials may be in need of a little calibration, but rest assured, you already have within you the raw materials to make it happen.

Calibrating Your Hunger Scale

To return to your roots and rediscover your brilliant, built-in feeding sensor, I'd like you to first visualize a scale from 0 to 5.

At levels 0 and 1, you are experiencing low blood sugar and feel very hungry, light-headed, weak, and even shaky. This is your body's way of warning you of its desperate need for sugar in the form of carbohydrates, which you already learned break down into sugar. You probably won't reach for celery sticks at this level because your body innately knows that celery won't be enough to boost blood sugar and make you feel better. You'll more likely find yourself elbow-deep in the cookie jar. I call this the loud level of hunger. It's sort of like that family member or friend we all know and love, who talks so loud they are virtually impossible to ignore.

When babies reach the level of loud hunger, they get very vocal, letting out a panic-stricken, blood-curdling scream to express their level of extreme discomfort. They may very well vomit near the end of the feeding because they guzzled so quickly, eating more than their little body could physically handle. This is far from a peaceful situation, isn't it? Just like babies, when we allow ourselves to reach this level of hunger, we always end up eating more than we physically need; therefore, it's always best to avoid this level in the first place.

Moving up the scale to levels 2 and 3, you will still feel hungry; however, the need for food isn't as urgent. It's what I call quiet hunger. Because you aren't in crisis mode, you can still function quite well and typically make more sound food choices. This is the most ideal time to eat because the chances of overeating are drastically reduced.

At levels 4 and 5, your body is relaxed, and you feel satisfied. Notice I didn't say "full." There is a difference between satisfied and full: Satisfied is how infants feel when they let go of the bottle or breast, while full is overly satisfied.

It helps to think of satisfied as eating until your stomach is two-thirds full. You want to leave a little room for the wonderful process of digestion to take place; if not, you will likely experience discomfort, gas, or heartburn.

Here is a visual guide of the scale to help you:

10— Stuffed (Thanksgiving Day full)
9— Overfull
8— Overfull
7— Full
6— Full
5— Satisfied (⅔ full)
4— Satisfied (⅔ full)
3— Quiet hunger
2— Quiet hunger
1— Loud hunger (empty)
0— Loud hunger (empty)

You will notice there are two levels assigned to each category of hunger/fullness. The difference between each level is subtle, yet significant. In each category, you will feel the effects of hunger more strongly at levels 0 and 2. Similarly, the effects of fullness will be more prominent at levels 5, 7, 9, and of course 10.

Once you become more in tune with your body, you will be able to recognize the difference between, say, a level 0 (I am ready to eat my arm) and a level 1 (I'm really hungry, but not enough to eat my arm.)

If we spend just a little more time eating to the level of satisfied, not only would we experience more physical and mental peace in our lives, we'd also have more energy and burn excess, unwanted fat. If you think about it, babies don't have to count calories to ensure they are getting enough to grow and thrive; they listen to their body, and it never fails them.

You can do the same. Because your body knows what it needs, it is, in a sense, its own calorie calculator. If you pay attention to what it's trying to tell you and put the fork down when it signals you are at a level 4 or 5, I promise you will shed excess fat if you have it to shed.

To help you practice your new style of eating, let's take this one step further. Pretend now that you were born with a built-in traffic light in your brain. When the light is green, you are experiencing either loud or quiet hunger. This is your cue to GO eat something. A yellow light means caution, signaling you to SLOW down, check in, and listen to what your body is trying to tell you. This is such an important signal, because if you miss it, you'll likely blow through the red STOP light and overeat. When the light turns red, you've reached a level 4 or 5, and it's time to put the fork down.

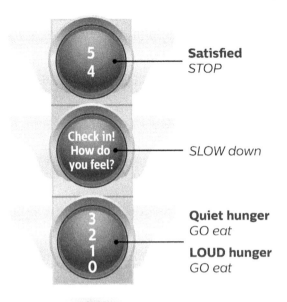

Traffic Light Hunger Scale

How Much Food Will It Take to Satisfy You?

So how much food does it take to reach a level 4 or 5, and how can you best ensure you don't overeat? The most effective suggestion I can offer you comes from the wisdom contained in Ayurvedic medicine.

Ayurveda, which translates into "the science of life," is an Indian healing system developed thousands of years ago. In Ayurveda, the optimum portion size to reach a level of satisfied is two cupped handfuls of food at every meal.

I know that doesn't sound like much, especially if you're used to eating a large plate of food for dinner every night, but give it a try at your next meal, and pay attention to how you feel. My guess is you will feel more satisfied than you think.

Here are a few questions to ask yourself if you still feel hungry after a meal:

1. Did my meal consist of mostly processed foods high in salt and sugar, with little or no Earthfoods? If so, it is likely your body is still searching for nutrients, which presents itself as hunger.

    Solution: Follow the guidelines for "How to Make a PeaceMeal" in Missing Peace #4 to ensure your meals contain plenty of satisfying, fiber-rich Earthfoods and healthy fats.

2. Am I well-hydrated? Even slight dehydration can be interpreted as hunger.

    Solution: Drink at least 8 oz. of water to see if it makes a difference.

3. Did I have a particularly active day today? When my day consists of going outside for a run in the morning and cleaning up the house in the afternoon, I can almost guarantee I will feel hungrier than usual, and the hunger sometimes doesn't strike until the next day.

Solution: Have another serving of roasted veggies or spoonful or two of quinoa pilaf at dinner, then seen how you feel.

Beyond Satisfied

Did you know your stomach has the capacity to stretch to accommodate up to an entire gallon of food? This, coupled with the fact that you are human, means that no matter how pure your intentions, there will be times when you eat beyond a level 5.

If you stop and think about it (and are really honest with yourself), you probably end most of your meals feeling beyond satisfied. Perhaps you eat to a level 6 or 7; on Thanksgiving, you may even reach a level 10. This is what I refer to as "Thanksgiving Day full," or a maximum capacity of one gallon.

I don't want you to feel bad about your past episodes of overeating because remember, you have strong roots. You were once a perfectly mindful baby with a very precise appetite scale. So wherever you are today on this spectrum, you are there because you trained your body to unlearn these early eating patterns.

For example, you may find that you regularly eat to a level 7 and therefore falsely believe this is satisfied, when in fact it is oversatisfied. Don't worry; all it takes is a little tweaking of your appetite scale to calibrate it back to your natural set point. The Make Peace exercise below will help you.

Make Peace Exercise: Return to Your Roots

1. Spend one full week tracking your level of hunger and fullness before and after each meal. The idea is not to judge yourself but to bring awareness to how much you are really eating. Use the scale below to help you.

   10— Stuffed (Thanksgiving Day full)
   9— Overfull
   8— Overfull
   7— Full
   6— Full
   5— Satisfied (⅔ full)
   4— Satisfied (⅔ full)
   3— Quiet hunger
   2— Quiet hunger
   1— Loud hunger (empty)
   0— Loud hunger (empty)

2. Return to your roots. Using the Traffic Light Hunger Scale tool to help you, start by choosing one meal that you will commit to consciously ending at a level 4–5, and do this for one week. Whether breakfast, lunch, or dinner, pay attention to your body, and eat until you are satisfied (or two-thirds full). To ensure success, don't allow your hunger to reach 0–1 (Loud Hunger). You will eat most mindfully at a Quiet Hunger level (level 2–3).

3. Strengthen your roots. Continue to build on your progress by adding a second meal to consciously end

at a level 4–5. Journal this experience by recording your sensations, both physical and emotional. How did you feel when you put the fork down at 4 or 5? Peaceful? Energized? Satisfied? Conflicted? Deprived?

Return to Your Light of Peace

Before taking your first bite of food, enter into a state of presence by taking a long, slow, deep breath in and letting it out. Tap into the strength of your Light of Peace, and allow it to reveal your true level of hunger, while placing full trust in your ability to sense how much your body really requires to be satisfied.

As you enjoy your meal, continue breathing into your Light of Peace while you taste every forkful. The more present you are, the easier it will be to recognize you've truly had enough to eat.

Recommended Peace of Health Shake

Healthy Brain Shake

7 Earthfood Servings ❤❤❤❤❤❤❤

12 oz. unsweetened almond, cashew, coconut, or flax milk
2 tbsp. Earthfood Powder
½ tbsp. MCT oil

⅛ cup walnuts
¼ of a small avocado, peeled and seeded
1 tbsp. fresh turmeric
2 cups fresh organic spinach or kale
½ cup frozen wild blueberries
¼ lemon with rind

Instructions:

Add all ingredients to a high-powered blender (such as Vitamix, Blendtec, or Ninja) in the order listed and blend until smooth.

Nutrition Facts: Calories: 460; Total Fat: 36 g; Saturated Fat: 9 g; Sodium: 490 mg; Potassium: 750 mg; Total Carbohydrates: 30 g; Dietary Fiber: 12 g; Net Carbohydrates: 18 g; Sugar: 7 g (no added sugar); Protein: 16 g

Note: Peace of Health shakes are not sweet, and that is by design. Sweetness is a trained preference, one that can be changed. The goal is to recalibrate your taste buds so that you begin to pick up the natural sweetness of the small amount of fruit in the shakes, without having to add sweetener or extra fruit. For a sweeter shake, refer to the tips offered in the "Do-It-Yourself Shakes" section at the beginning of the book.

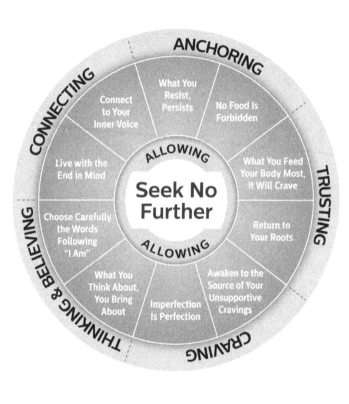

Chapter 4: Craving

Missing Peace #6: Awaken to the Source of Your Unsupportive Cravings
Missing Peace #7: Imperfection Is Perfection

You are now ready to journey further around the Path to Peace and learn how to navigate unsupportive cravings that seem to creep up without warning.

Your higher self only knows wellness. When you disturb it by overindulging in harmful substances, foods, or behaviors, it will give you a warning signal to adjust your thoughts and habits. Missing Peace #6: Awaken to the Source of Your Unsupportive Cravings will help you gain a better understanding of the origin of these cravings, along with steps you can take to stay in control.

Missing Peace #7: Imperfection Is Perfection reminds you that you are, in fact, a perfectly imperfect human being; therefore, striving for 100 percent perfection in your food choices is 100 percent unrealistic. Here, you are encouraged to give yourself permission to be perfectly imperfect and reframe how you approach food cravings. As a guide, I offer a plan to successfully honor your cravings in a healthier, more peaceful way.

Missing Peace #6: Awaken to the Source of Your Unsupportive Cravings

> We love salt, fat and sugar. We're hard-wired
> to go for those flavors. They trip our dopamine
> networks, which are our craving networks.
> —Michael Pollan

Have you ever felt the overwhelming urge to dig into a bag of potato chips? I know I have. Sometimes, the desire stems from a physical craving for salt and crunch, while other times, it is brought on by stress, such as a tight work deadline or family health crisis.

Food cravings can be both mental and physical in nature, and this Missing Peace will identify several of them. But first, what exactly do I mean by unsupportive cravings? And is there such a thing as a supportive craving?

Unsupportive food cravings are those caused by certain food substances (e.g., sugar and artificial sweeteners) and emotional states (e.g., stress).

A supportive food craving is your body physically calling out for a food that will supply it with vitamins or minerals it's lacking (or for water to reverse a state of dehydration). It generally drives good health and attempts to return the body to homeostasis or balance.

For example, craving vegetables (and thus eating them) will serve to nourish your body with essential vitamins, minerals, and antioxidants. Although typically thought of as unsupportive, craving salt can be supportive when it results from significant sweat loss (and therefore sodium loss) after a five-mile run in 80 degree weather. These cravings are your body's way of trying to restore inner balance.

In my experience, there are several factors that can trigger unsupportive food cravings, binges, and overeating. These periods of overeating can feel almost like an out-of-body experience, where you watch what's going on and yet can't stop. The factors include sugar, salt, and fat in processed food; dehydration; poor gut health; leptin resistance; artificial sweeteners; alcohol; head-hunger; and lack of sleep.

Let's start with the first of these: sugar, salt, and fat in processed food.

Sugar, Salt, and Fat in Processed Food

Understand that the sugar, salt, and fat I'm referring to is the type found in highly processed foods, such as sugary treats and beverages; refined, white flour products like bread, pasta, pretzels, and crackers; frozen meals; and fried foods swimming in unhealthy fats. I'm not talking about the natural sugars found in Earthfoods like fruits and vegetables, or healthy fats in avocados, nuts, and seeds. These nutrient-rich foods are loaded with antioxidants and play a key role in healing the body by reducing inflammation. They also carry natural fibers along with them, which serve to weaken their effect on blood sugar.

Not long ago, I attended a gluten-free expo in Chicago. Exhibiting were countless gluten-free food vendors, offering up samples of their special products. If you're not familiar, gluten is the protein found in wheat, rye, and barley and processed food products containing these ingredients, such as bread, cereal, pasta, pancakes, pizza, and other high-sugar, low-nutrition foods.

Gluten causes a whole spectrum of problems for many people, ranging from non-celiac gluten sensitivity (NCGS) to celiac disease (an autoimmune condition where ingestion of gluten leads to damage in the small intestine, creating iron deficiency anemia, joint pain, depression, anxiety, fatigue, and migraines).

According to the Celiac Disease Foundation, some people experience symptoms of celiac disease, such as foggy mind, depression, ADHD-like behavior, abdominal pain, bloating, diarrhea, constipation, headaches, bone or joint pain, and chronic fatigue, when they have gluten in their diet, but they do not test positive for celiac disease. NCGS is generally used to refer to this condition; removing gluten from the diet resolves symptoms.

As you can probably imagine, the exhibiting vendors at the gluten-free expo were not featuring naturally gluten-free foods like fresh produce, nuts, seeds, fresh meats, and seafood. Rather, it was like walking through a processed food emporium. The first day of the convention, I walked around to check out all of the booths and found everything from doughnuts to pizza to frosted cupcakes to coffee cake.

One day, I was unprepared. Being away from home, I wasn't armed with my usual Earthfood fare: my morning smoothie and other staples typically found in my meals, such as raw vegetables and nuts, salmon, and fruit. Did I mention I was hungry?

Even though I had full faith in my ability to stay on course, as I shuffled through the aisles, my hunger got the best of me, and I broke down and sampled a few crackers. Next up: chocolate chip cookies, a doughnut, and a slice of pizza. In between were corn chips, granola, and a snack bar. I lost track of how many samples I garbaged down, and the bizarre part was that I didn't feel the least bit satisfied. Sure, I was bloated but not nourished. I was in a foggy zone of temporary food addiction; had I not felt so crappy, I'm sure I would've kept on to the next booth.

I was depressed; after all, I was supposed to be a pro at this. My days of glutinous binging were far behind me, weren't they?

This eerily familiar feeling was one I experienced on a daily basis for three years when I suffered from binge eating disorder. It scared me to the core because the last time I visited that dark and lonely place was August of 2000, my final binge in Las Vegas.

So what triggered this out-of-control behavior? At first, I wanted to blame it on a lack of willpower, but that didn't make sense. How could I have possessed such strong willpower for sixteen years, only for it to instantaneously go up in smoke in one single day? The magic formula was a combination of processed sugar, salt, and fat, which collectively work to make food hyperpalatable and virtually irresistible.

Sugar, in particular, is an addictive substance. The more you eat it, the more you crave it. And if you aren't used to eating it, the effects are much more intense. For me, I literally felt it in my brain and joints the day after the gluten-free expo. My brain was foggy, and my body ached.

Besides creating an inflammatory environment in the body, sugar causes rapid spikes in your blood sugar, which forces your body to produce the hormone insulin in an effort to sweep up the sugar and store it in your cells. This entire process is by design. It's what a normal, healthy, and vibrant body is supposed to do. The problem is, when you eat more sugar (and thus produce more insulin), your body responds with heightened hunger, decreased metabolism, and increased fat storage.

Yes, since insulin is a fat-storage hormone, the more of it you force your body to produce, the higher the likelihood you will store excess fat. I'm sure this isn't something you bargain for when you set out to drink that fancy, sugar-sweetened coffee beverage, is it?

Compounding these effects in the body is the fact that the sugar, salt, and fat found in packaged and processed foods, like chocolate ice cream and potato chips, is biologically addictive.

Dr. David Katz, director of Yale University's Prevention Research Center, says,[3]

> Our attraction to sweets and salt, carbohydrates and fat is hardwired from the Stone Age. Back then, food cravings were reliable signals to our ancestors to seek out certain foods that would provide energy (sugar, fat) and essential minerals (salt). Today, food is plentiful and it's easy to avoid physical activity, but we've preserved craving tendencies because evolution is very slow.

It also doesn't help that the simple act of eating salty, fatty, or sugary foods triggers your brain to release opioids and dopamine—both feel-good chemicals that actually compel you to overeat. So you see, frequent consumption of calorie-dense, processed foods may alter your brain responses in a way that makes you eat more.

Dehydration

Did you know that thirst can be mistaken for hunger in your body? All too often, we find ourselves reaching for a snack, when what we really need is a glass of water. How can you tell the difference? Drink a glass of water, and if the hunger pangs go away, then you know it was thirst.

To avoid this false hunger, be sure to drink plenty of water throughout the day—enough to produce urine that is pale

---

[3] Dana Sullivan Kilroy, "Cravings Could Be Defeated with Two Little Words," *Los Angeles Times,* July 21, 2012.

yellow in color and almost clear. Keep in mind that once you begin feeling thirsty, your body is already dehydrated. So don't wait until you get to that point.

Poor Gut Health

You might find it hard to believe that the bacteria living in your gut outnumber the cells of your body by a factor of ten to one. This collection of more than a hundred trillion organisms living within your intestines, called your microbiome, influences practically everything about you.

Typically, when we think of bacteria on our body, we immediately have the urge to break out a bottle of hand sanitizer. Not so fast. Not all bacteria are bad; in fact, many are beneficial to your health, and destroying them is the worst thing you could do.

When the healthy, beneficial bacteria are thriving in our microbiome, we tend to experience better overall health and well-being, including

- a better mood,
- a stronger immune system,
- a lower risk of disease,
- improved quality of sleep,
- healthy digestion,
- healthy body weight, and
- healthy food cravings.

So what does bacteria have to do with food cravings and overeating? When the wrong bacteria have control of our gut, they can dictate what we eat by inducing food cravings, making us prefer junk food over Earthfood.

Researchers are just scratching the surface on how influential some bacteria truly are. For example, these bacteria can release toxins in response to certain foods. These toxins will make us feel good when we eat something they like and not so good when they disagree with our food choices. But this doesn't mean that the foods they prefer are the ones that are actually good for us.[4]

I know this may sound hopeless, but don't worry; you can actually manipulate your gut bacteria to ensure the survival and growth of good bacteria and therefore induce healthy food cravings.

The key is twofold: to fuel your body with foods that populate good bacteria and minimize those foods that can destroy them in favor of the bad ones.

Remember what I said about the power of your body to crave what it is fed most? Can you now begin to see how these cravings have much to do with the health of your microbiome?

To grow and sustain the good bacteria, in addition to eating a balanced diet chock-full of a wide variety of Earthfoods

---

[4] David Williams, "Gut Bacteria May Influence Food Cravings."

and low in processed foods, you'll also want to eat a steady supply of probiotic and prebiotic-rich foods.

Probiotics are foods or supplements containing live bacteria that replace or add to the beneficial bacteria normally present in your gut. They include fermented foods such as plain yogurt, kefir, kombucha, kvass, natto, raw sauerkraut and pickles, miso, kimchi, tempeh, and raw, unfiltered apple cider vinegar. In addition to eating fermented foods every day, I also recommend taking a good quality probiotic supplement.

In general, a quality probiotic supplement will contain at least ten different probiotic strains and fifteen billion colony forming units. You will also want to ensure the probiotic guarantees potency, meaning the microbes are alive when you take it. Some supplements guarantee a live microbe count at the time of manufacture, but this doesn't mean that amount is alive when you ingest it.

Prebiotics are food for the good bacteria and are just as important as probiotics. They include nuts and vegetables such as asparagus, leeks, artichokes, garlic, carrots, peas, beans, onions, chicory, jicama, broccoli, tomatoes, cauliflower, spinach, kale, and chard, and fresh or frozen fruits, like bananas, cherries, apples, pears, oranges, strawberries, cranberries, blueberries, blackberries, raspberries, and kiwi.

Personally, I take a few steps each day to make sure I'm keeping the good bugs alive and growing in my body. First, I take a probiotic supplement every morning. I follow that up with a nice hot cup of water with 1 tbsp. of Bragg apple cider vinegar mixed in. For breakfast, I add prebiotic-rich frozen blueberries and fresh kale to my smoothie. I end my day with another cup of hot water and apple cider vinegar. In between, I chow down on several servings of veggies, nuts, and seeds to get me through the day.

Step 2 in populating a healthy microbiome is to minimize those foods, substances, and habits that can destroy good bacteria, including exposure to pesticides, smoking, and foods with artificial food coloring, refined sugar, and artificial sweeteners. In addition, overuse of antibiotics and hand sanitizers is a problem, as they kill off both bad and good bacteria.

Leptin Resistance

When you eat a meal, you expect to feel satisfied. But what if that doesn't happen? What if you never feel full? What if your hunger pangs don't disappear? What if you feel the urge to snack all day long?

Setting out on a journey to healthier eating is a beautiful thing, but the motivation to continue often fizzles out. And it's not because you stopped caring about yourself, but rather, your body feels hungry, and your cravings are out of control.

When I was suffering from binge eating disorder, I never felt full. And I mean never. It didn't matter how much I ate; my body always wanted to keep on eating. This was a foreign feeling to me, one I couldn't wrap my head around.

Then I learned about leptin, a little hormone produced by our fat cells. It's a pretty powerful hormone too, one that controls your appetite by regulating brain cells that tell you how much to eat. It also plays a role in weight control.

In a nutshell, leptin tells the brain that we have plenty of fat stored, which sends the signal to stop eating. Low levels of leptin tell the brain we are at risk of starvation, and hunger and cravings kick in.

Where this whole system goes a bit haywire is when leptin is produced in ample amounts but the brain doesn't see it, creating a condition called leptin resistance.

So what does this really mean? The brain mistakenly thinks it's starving and therefore turns on the signal to eat more and expend less, creating the perfect environment for weight gain, and making it nearly impossible to shed body fat. What's worse, the very process of losing weight reduces leptin, so your brain attempts to hold on to body fat by increasing appetite and hunger, while decreasing metabolism. How frustrating.

This invisible, vicious cycle is likely why we blame ourselves for lacking willpower. It has nothing to do with willpower; it's your body biologically calling out for food.

If what you just read sounds like a carbon copy of your struggles with weight loss and food cravings, please know it's not your fault. Diets high in sugar (particularly fructose) and processed foods promote surges of leptin, which over time can create leptin resistance. These diets also compromise the integrity of the gut, leading to an overgrowth of bad bacteria.

To regulate leptin, you must get back to the basics. This means filling your plate with Earthfoods, such as vegetables, fruits, nuts, seeds, and avocados, and healthy fats like coconut and olive oil, and also including a moderate amount of high-quality protein, such as organic free-range eggs, wild salmon, and grass-fed beef.

A daily dose of probiotic-rich foods and supplements is also necessary to keep the good bugs growing and the bad ones at bay. Remember that what you feed your body most, it will crave.

You deserve to have the craving needle move in a favorable direction, so stop counting calories and start putting the good, whole foods in; before you know it, you'll be begging for broccoli over burgers. Really.

Artificial Sweeteners

Two pink packets in my already-sweetened bowl of maple and brown sugar-flavored oatmeal. Diet Pepsi with nearly every meal. Diet yogurts and pudding cups for snacks, and sugar-free gum when I wasn't eating a meal or snack. It makes me shudder every time I think of all the chemicals I poured into my body. It's no wonder it was confused, feeling hungry, craving sugar, and riddled with constant headaches. These are just some of the side effects that can occur on a steady diet of artificial sweeteners.

You see, many people falsely believe they are saving calories when they opt for the light, 100-calorie yogurt, sweetened with aspartame, instead of indulging in the plain, full-fat version. This couldn't be further from the truth.

Studies continuously reveal the dark side of artificial sweeteners, namely aspartame (Equal and Nutrasweet), acesulfame potassium (Sunnet and Sweet One), saccharin (Sugar Twin and Sweet 'n' Low), and sucralose (Splenda).

Did you know that sweetness—whether from sugar or artificial sweeteners—enhances the appetite and motivation to eat? Also, because they are hundreds of times sweeter than regular white table sugar, artificial sweeteners encourage sugar cravings and sugar dependence.[5]

If I had my way, artificial sweeteners wouldn't exist.

I can read your mind: *But Melanie, what about stevia?* Stevia is a plant grown in South America that has been used for centuries as a natural sweetener and health remedy. Of the three categories of stevia on the market today (green leaf stevia, stevia extracts, and highly processed stevia or white powder), green leaf stevia is by far the best option because it is the closest to nature and the form touted for its health benefits. It is literally the stevia plant ground up into a powder, making it the least processed form.

I choose not to use stevia because just like artificial sweeteners, it causes me to crave sugar. If you use stevia or

---

[5] Yang, "Gain Weight by 'Going Diet'?"

eat foods sweetened with it, this is something you may want to consider.

Since I removed artificial sweeteners all those years ago, I feel more in tune with my body. I no longer crave sugar like a drug, and my appetite and hunger are real, not governed by chemicals.

Knowledge is power, but what you do with that knowledge will impact your health in ways you never imagined. I'd like you to think of it this way: artificial sweeteners are synthetic chemicals; they aren't natural, and they certainly don't act naturally in your body.

Alcohol

It never fails; I have one too many glasses of wine (and for me, the magic number is two), and the next day, I feel the need to eat everything in sight. My body never seems to crave its usual smoothie or leafy green salad, but rather it demands processed snack foods, especially salty tortilla chips. I gravitate to the pantry like a magnet to a refrigerator and proceed to eat half of the bag.

This day-after-drinking indulgence always frustrated me, until I learned there was a biological reason for it. As it turns out, alcohol in any form decreases blood sugar levels, temporarily and overnight. Low blood sugar is a signal to kick up hunger. And because it's also a diuretic, drinking alcohol causes you to pee more. If you're not consciously rehydrating with plenty of water, dehydration sets in, which your body misinterprets as hunger. Talk about a double-whammy.

And if that's not bad enough, because your liver is heavily involved in the process of detoxifying your body to remove the alcohol, it is unable to carry out the important job of releasing stored sugar to counteract falling blood sugar. What happens as a result? You guessed it: insatiable hunger.

Because I wasn't willing to give up red wine, I knew a few strategies were in order if I wanted to have my wine and drink it too. This three-step plan is like my own little insurance policy against overindulging on the wrong foods the next day.

1. Never drink on an empty stomach. I usually take my first sip of wine after I've eaten about a quarter of my dinner. This little trick prevents the blood sugar plunge that happens when alcohol hits your system without any food to slow it down.
2. To ensure I don't get dehydrated, I always drink 8–16 oz. of water with my glass of wine.
3. Limit myself to one, 8-oz. glass of wine per night. Even though a true portion of wine is 5 oz., I secretly feel cheated by such a small amount, so I decided to create my own version of a portion. For your information, the following are standard portion sizes for alcohol:

   a. beer: 12 oz.
   b. wine (red or white): 5 oz.
   c. hard liquor: 1.5 oz.

Head-Hunger

Have you ever felt the strong urge to tear open a bag of chips after hearing some unexpected bad news? Upon sitting down at your desk to begin a dreaded work project, do you sometimes swear you hear the chocolate chip cookies from the office vending machine calling your name? Did you find yourself elbow-deep in a carton of strawberry ice cream immediately following the last argument you had with your partner?

You're not alone.

Confession: I tend to procrastinate. In fact, some would call me a master procrastinator. If I'm faced with a task before me that I'm not looking forward to, you can bet I will get a sudden urge to scoop the cat's litter box or clean out the refrigerator.

If you ever use food to cope with life or find yourself eating when you aren't physically hungry, you are most certainly feeding your head-hunger. Maybe you eat when you're bored, stressed, sad, angry, depressed, or happy; whatever the reason, this is a sure sign of disconnect.

When was the last time you witnessed a baby cry because he needed a diaper change, and Mom came running with a bottle? She tries to feed him, but he keeps crying. If he could talk, he'd probably say, "Hey, dummy, check the diaper. I'm wet and uncomfortable, not hungry." He's upset but doesn't turn to food to ease his emotions because he knows it won't work.

The strong urge to eat in response to head-hunger is a way of attempting to avoid a situation or emotion that you don't want to face head-on. I admire babies, for they are the most brilliant eaters of all. Whatever the situation, they deal with it in the most appropriate and natural way possible. It's what they instinctively and innately know to be the only way. The only time it makes sense for them to eat is when they are physically hungry.

Don't forget: you used to be that baby.

If head-hunger only happened once in a while, there would be no cause for concern. But the reality is, it's usually an automatic habit, embedded in your behavior, possibly since childhood. It is what you know and are comfortable with. In fact, it would feel weird to *not* eat.

If your loving, well-meaning mother always soothed your scraped knee with a kiss and a lollipop, to this day, you may immediately turn to a bowl of candy when you have any sort of ache or pain.

The next time you find yourself stressed out and ready to dig into a plate of double chocolate brownies, first bring awareness to the situation you are facing by taking a long, slow, deep breath in and out. Awareness is like turning on a light in a pitch-black room; there's no way to know it's there if you can't see it.

Second, speak to the emotion by saying, either out loud or to yourself, "I see you, stress."

Third, I'd like you to dig a little deeper and turn up the intensity of that light to uncover the source of this emotion. Why exactly do you feel stressed? Did you just check your bank account balance, only to discover that there isn't enough money to cover your mortgage this month? What you're doing here is bringing even more awareness to the situation. Speak to your stress again; call it out by saying, "I see you, stress, and I know why you are here."

Finally, it's time to face the emotion or situation head-on. In other words, rip off that bandage and really feel it. It's extremely important at this stage to go within and connect with the real you.

Take a few slow, deep breaths, sit with the feeling for a moment (I promise, it won't kill you), and ask yourself, What action is my higher self guiding me to take right now? The answer will come to you very naturally, just like it does a baby, and you will know immediately that it's the right one because you will feel a sense of peace wash over you. This is your indication that you have connected to the larger part of you.

When I'm facing a bout of procrastination and take myself through the above exercise, the answer that usually comes to me is, "I really need to meditate." It works every time.

As you ponder over the solution I just offered, it's really important that you understand one simple truth: You always have a choice. You can choose to eat; after all, it's your right. Think back to Missing Peace #2: What You Resist, Persists. If you tell yourself you can't eat in response to an unfavorable situation, you are only giving power to the act of eating, and I'll bet you end up eating, a lot.

Shine a bright light on your head-hunger by answering these four questions:

1. What is the emotion or situation I am wanting to feed? (e.g., stress)
2. Why do I feel this way? (e.g., I'm overwhelmed with end-of-the-month projects at work)
3. What action is my higher self guiding me to take right now? (e.g., To practice deep breathing exercises)
4. A confirming question: How did I deal with this emotion or situation as a baby?

Lack of Sleep

If you want a voracious appetite and insatiable cravings, then all you have to do is skimp on sleep.

But what constitutes enough sleep? According to the National Sleep Foundation, it's between seven and nine hours per night. I can't even begin to tell you the number of people who laugh out loud when I share this recommendation. "Yeah right, Melanie. I'm lucky if I get five hours of sleep," they retort, followed up with, "Besides, I feel perfectly fine on that amount." *That's even worse*, I think silently to myself.

Due to a genetic mutation, only 1 percent of the population can get by on less than seven hours of sleep each night. And

I can almost guarantee that you aren't a member of this special club.

So how exactly does lack of sleep affect appetite and food cravings? When your body is in a sleep-deprived state, it experiences increased levels of the hormone ghrelin, which stimulates the appetite. This means if you sleep less than seven hours a night, you will eat more, and I'm not talking carrot sticks and cucumber slices. Chips, candy, and other high-calorie foods become simply irresistible when you're lacking sleep.

Repeat after me: Sleep is not a luxury, it's a necessity. In fact, it's the most important thing you can do for your well-being.

Make Peace Exercise: Take Charge of Your Cravings

1. Spend one week contemplating the sources of your unsupportive cravings. Really pay attention to what you feel is driving these cravings, and then assign a number to the strength of each below. A rating of 1 indicates a very weak link, whereas a score of 5 is very strong.

    a. Sugar: _____
    b. Dehydration: _____
    c. Poor gut health: _____
    d. Leptin resistance: _____
    e. Artificial sweeteners: _____
    f. Alcohol: _____

     g.   Head-hunger: _____

     h.   Lack of sleep: _____

2. Any of the above sources that you rated a 3 (or above) deserves some attention. Choose the one that speaks to you most and allow your higher self to formulate a realistic plan that will work for you. Then put your plan into immediate action. For example, if you assigned "Lack of sleep" a score of 4, your plan may look something like this: "I will turn off the television thirty minutes earlier than usual, making my new bedtime 10:30 p.m."

Once you've made this plan a habit, you can choose to continue making improvements in this particular area if needed (by gradually getting more sleep until you reach seven hours), or formulate a plan for your next high-scoring source.

Your plan:

I will:

_____

_____

_____

_____

_____

_____

_____

_____

_____

_____

_____

_____

Return to Your Light of Peace

When faced with an unsupportive craving, stop, close your eyes, and take a long, slow, deep breath in and out to return to your Light of Peace. You are now in the present moment and in harmony your higher self. Ask yourself, What is the source of this unsupportive craving? Wait for the answer, and as you continue to breathe, ask, What can I do to bring my body back into a state of peace and well-being?

Recommended Peace of Health Shake

Gut-Loving Chocolate Peanut Butter Shake

5 Earthfood Servings ♥ ♥ ♥ ♥ ♥

2 oz. plain, whole milk kefir (if dairy-intolerant, omit and use a total of 10 oz. of unsweetened nut milk instead)
8 oz. unsweetened almond, cashew, coconut, or flax milk
2 tbsp. Earthfood Powder
1 tbsp. raw cacao powder
1 tbsp. fresh ground peanut butter
1 tsp. pure vanilla extract
½ banana, ripe (frozen makes it creamier)
¼ of a small avocado, peeled and seeded

Instructions:

Add all ingredients to a high-powered blender (such as Vitamix, Blendtec, or Ninja) in the order listed and blend until smooth.

Nutrition Facts: Calories: 435; Total Fat: 29 g; Saturated Fat: 10 g; Sodium: 250 mg; Potassium: 450 mg; Total Carbohydrates: 32 g; Dietary Fiber: 11 g; Net Carbohydrates: 21 g; Sugar: 10 g (no added sugar); Protein: 17 g

Note: Peace of Health shakes are not sweet, and that is by design. Sweetness is a trained preference, one that can be changed. The goal is to recalibrate your taste buds so that you begin to pick up the natural sweetness of the small amount of fruit in the shakes, without having to add sweetener or extra fruit. For a sweeter shake, refer to the tips offered in the "Do-It-Yourself Shakes" section at the beginning of the book.

Missing Peace #7: Imperfection Is Perfection

> If you can't see anything beautiful about
> yourself, get a better mirror.
> —Shane Koyczan

There is something unsettling about a diet full of only healthy food. It's like the body craves a little bit of fun every once in a while. I consider myself to be a pretty healthy eater: tons of veggies and greens, plenty of healthy fats, and probiotic-rich foods like kefir and fermented vegetables.

Because I feed my body this way, it craves these foods most often. However, at least a few times each week, my body also craves sweet and salt. This used to frustrate me to no end, because if my body is supposed to crave what I feed it most, and I feed it a healthy diet, why in the heck do I crave chocolate and tortilla chips if I don't eat them regularly?

Then I was introduced to the works of Dr. David Katz. If you recall from Missing Peace #6: Awaken to the Source of Your Unsupportive Cravings, it was Dr. Katz who said the following: "Our attraction to sweets and salt, carbohydrates and fat is hardwired from the Stone Age." This helped me to remember that I am, in fact, human, and even though I eat nutritious food 90 percent of the time, human beings crave certain foods and tastes by nature. Therefore, an expectation of 100 percent is unrealistic; actually, it's completely ridiculous. So I decided to reframe the way I approach my cravings:

"Hello, my name is Melanie Jatsek, and I crave sugar and salt from time to time, which therefore makes me a perfectly imperfect human being."

Boy, does that feel good. Talk about a total sense of inner freedom. I encourage you to give yourself permission to be a perfectly imperfect human being. Shout it from the rooftops. Embrace it.

I often chuckle when I run into someone I know at the grocery store. The encounter goes something like this: We exchange a warm, friendly greeting, and then she proceeds to apologize for the contents of her grocery cart, blaming the box of cookies on her husband and children. After I assure her it's okay, I then point to the chocolates in my cart. So if I ever run into you at the grocery store, and you happen to have a food in your cart that you're not proud of, instead of hiding it or explaining it away, stand proud and repeat my mantra:

"Hello, my name is _____, and I crave _____ and _____ from time to time, which therefore makes me a perfectly imperfect human being!"

How can you strike a healthy balance between wholesome, nutritious food and a little fun? A genuine concern for many is being able to have our cake and eat it too, without going over the deep end and eating the entire cake. Let's face it: it's a bit unrealistic to have your trigger food in the house and not expect to eat it.

Four Steps to Honor Your Cravings in a Healthier Way

I have found a way to successfully honor my cravings in a healthier way, and I think you'll find it works for you too. Here's what to do:

Step 1: Describe Your Craving

First, ask yourself, What is my body really craving right now? Describe your cravings using adjectives versus nouns, or specific foods. The reason for this is that most of the time, a craving can be satisfied by a healthier food offering the exact same properties you are craving, without perpetuating continued eating. It cures the craving and nourishes the body, all at the same time.

For example, are you in the mood for something

- creamy,
- crunchy,
- fizzy,
- salty,
- spicy, or
- sweet?

Step 2: Grant Permission

Next, even though I've just prompted you to describe your cravings with adjectives, you may still have a specific food in mind that you want to eat. In this step, I want you to give yourself full permission to eat the food you are craving, whether it's a doughnut, potato chips, or an ice cream sundae. This mental clearing puts you in control and releases the sex appeal of your trigger food.

An important point to note here is this: if what you are craving is your kryptonite food, and you can't control yourself around it, it's best not to have it in your house at all.

Step 3: Honor Your Craving

After giving yourself full permission to eat the food you are craving, it's time to feed your body what it really desires: fat, crunch, fizz, salt, spice, or sweet. It doesn't matter how these cravings are delivered, so why not aim for a choice that will honor your beautiful body?

For example, the other day, I arrived home sweaty and thirsty after a long, invigorating run in the park. After drinking a glass of water and taking a nice long, cool shower, I ventured into the kitchen in search of something salty. This made total sense because I just lost a lot of sodium in my sweat, so naturally my body delivered a salt craving to replenish it.

My first inclination was to open the pantry and grab the bag of tortilla chips, which I've done countless times in the past and always end up eating half of the bag, if not more. With one hand on a bag of Garden of Eatin' Red Hot Blues tortilla chips, I stopped, took a breath, and then asked myself, What is my body really craving right now? I discovered that what I really desired was salt and crunch, which the chips offer so beautifully.

I thought about a better option, one that would not only satisfy these cravings but also help me stay in control and committed to my health goals, a food that would offer me peace instead of conflict. I landed on hummus, which offered 300 milligrams of sodium per serving. Salt craving: check. Now I needed something to quench my longing for crunch. I opted for some raw celery sticks and baby carrots. I am happy to report that my craving was perfectly satisfied, and I had no urge to continue eating.

The key to success in step 3 is to make sure your kitchen is stocked with healthier alternatives. Let's get real here: We both know if you are on a serious mission for salt and crunch, and the only food in your kitchen to deliver those qualities is a bag of chips, no matter how pure your intentions, you will not get in your car and drive to the store for hummus and carrots. You just won't.

Here are some foods to help you bust through your cravings in a healthier, more peaceful way:

Salty/Crunchy

- jicama sticks with fresh ground almond butter
- hard-boiled egg sprinkled with a shake or two of sea salt
- handful of raw, salted pumpkin seeds or pistachios
- hummus with celery sticks, red pepper strips, or baby carrots
- roasted broccoli, brussels sprouts, or cauliflower sprinkled with sea salt
- 3–4 Kalamata olives
- spoonful or two of fermented vegetables (kimchi or sauerkraut)
- roasted chickpeas seasoned with sea salt
- sprouted tortilla chips

Sweet

- a square or two of dark chocolate (72 percent cacao or higher)
- nutrition bar (<8 grams of sugar per serving and no artificial sweeteners)
- raw chocolate and strawberries

- apple slices drizzled with fresh ground peanut or almond butter and sprinkled with a tablespoon of dark chocolate chips and organic, unsweetened shredded coconut
- 2–3 pitted dates
- baked apple
- homemade trail mix: organic unsweetened coconut flakes + raw nuts + dark chocolate chips + sliced dates, dried wild blueberries, or goji berries

Creamy

- mashed avocado on sprouted bread
- 1 tbsp. of fresh ground almond butter, peanut butter, or cashew butter
- guacamole with raw veggies

Fizzy

- club soda or sparkling water with a twist of lemon (add 1 oz. of fresh squeezed orange or grapefruit juice for more flavor)
- kombucha

Spicy

- baked kale chips with a dash of cayenne pepper
- a spoonful or two of kimchi
- roasted chickpeas seasoned with cayenne pepper

Step 4: Evaluate Your Craving

Now it's time to evaluate whether your food craving was satisfied or not. The good news is, 99 percent of time, healthier alternatives will do the trick. But what happens when they don't? Then go ahead and give yourself full, guilt-free, nonjudgmental permission to drive to the store and settle your craving once and for all. This is the beauty of being a perfectly imperfect human being.

The Rule of 20

Since we are in fact perfectly imperfect human beings, doesn't it stand to reason that we should give ourselves permission to be imperfect with our daily food choices?

I have found that part of being a responsible adult requires honoring not only my health but also my humanness. This is why I never expect 100 percent in my eating and exercise habits. In fact, I believe 100 percent is unnatural for us humans, and we tend to rebel against it by quietly sabotaging our unrealistic expectations with an extra glass of wine or slice of pizza.

What if, instead, you made room for your humanness by building imperfection into your daily routine? This is where the Rule of 20 comes in.

Every morning, right after you open your eyes, I want you to declare that today will be a perfectly imperfect day. Lower your expectations. Take a deep breath and promise yourself, first, that you will fuel your body with healthy food because you deserve it.

Second, vow to cut yourself some slack and reserve 20 percent of your choices for that human side of you. For example, my 20 percent is reserved for one or two of the following treats: a glass of wine with dinner, an ounce or two of real cheese, a piece of high-quality chocolate, or pesto sauce for dipping my veggies.

The amazing part about the Rule of 20—besides the fact that it offers me a sense of freedom and liberation—is that I find I don't always take it. I may only have a glass of wine and cheese three nights a week and chocolate only four nights, but it's there if I want it. This built-in permission makes all the difference in the world.

Can't you feel the peace wash over your body as you imagine life where imperfection is not only embraced but also encouraged?

Whatever you do, don't forget to live. A slice of cake on your birthday, a warm doughnut from your favorite bakery, a cheeseburger and fries eaten while vacationing with your family—these are all part of living a peaceful life. Fear not.

If you are living from a place of honoring your body, these little celebrations and trips off of your normal, healthy path will not lead you astray. I promise that you will continue to remain at peace.

Make Peace Exercise: Be Perfectly Imperfect

Every morning for the next seven days, build imperfection into your day with the following morning declaration. Then, as you go about your day, pay close attention to your food cravings. When one strikes, follow the four-step plan below to honor it in a healthier way:

Your Morning Declaration

Every morning when you first wake up, declare that today is going to be a perfectly imperfect day. Take a deep breath and make the following promise to yourself: "Today I will honor my body by feeding it wholesome food, while respecting and making space for my humanness."

Honoring Your Cravings

1. Describe your craving: When a craving strikes, take a step back and ask yourself, What is my body really craving right now? Is it something creamy, crunchy, fizzy, salty, spicy, or sweet?
2. Grant permission: Take a deep breath and give yourself full permission to eat the food you are really craving.
3. Honor your craving: Quench that craving with a more wholesome alternative. Make a list of your go-to peaceful craving foods:

Crunchy: _____

Creamy: _____

Fizzy: _____

Salty: _____

Spicy: _____

Sweet: _____

4. Evaluate your craving: Was your craving satisfied by the healthier alternative? If not, give yourself unconditional permission to drive to the store and get the real thing.

Return to Your Light of Peace:

Make space for your humanness. Instead of fighting a food craving, be present for it. Take a moment to pause and turn inward to align with your higher self. Take a deep breath in and out, and surround yourself with your Light of Peace. Ask yourself, How can I honor this craving in the most peaceful way? Remember, you are loved, no matter what.

Recommended Peace of Health Shake

Berry Power Shake

6 Earthfood Servings ❤❤❤❤❤❤

12 oz. unsweetened almond, cashew, coconut, or flax milk
2 tbsp. Earthfood Powder

1 tbsp. chia seeds

¼ small avocado, peeled and seeded

½ tbsp. coconut butter

½ tbsp. fresh ground almond butter

¼ lemon with rind

½ cup frozen wild blueberries

½ cup frozen cranberries

Instructions:

Add all ingredients to a high-powered blender (such as Vitamix, Blendtec, or Ninja) in the order listed and blend until smooth.

Nutrition Facts: Calories: 440; Total Fat: 31 g; Saturated Fat: 7 g; Sodium: 460 mg; Potassium: 700 mg; Total Carbohydrates: 35 g; Dietary Fiber: 20 g; Net Carbohydrates: 15 g; Sugar: 9 g (no added sugar); Protein: 16 g

Note: Peace of Health shakes are not sweet, and that is by design. Sweetness is a trained preference, one that can be changed. The goal is to recalibrate your taste buds so that you begin to pick up the natural sweetness of the small amount of fruit in the shakes, without having to add sweetener or extra fruit. For a sweeter shake, refer to the tips offered in the "Do-It-Yourself Shakes" section at the beginning of the book.

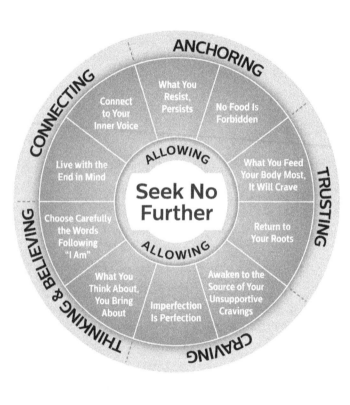

Chapter 5: Thinking and Believing

Missing Peace #8: What You Think about, You Bring About
Missing Peace #9: Choose Carefully the Words Following "I Am"

In this phase of your Path to Peace, you are taken on an inner journey and asked to explore your thoughts, beliefs, and self-talk. Although you were introduced to the power of your mind in the Anchoring phase, in Missing Peace #8: What You Think about, You Bring About, you will dig even deeper to uncover and make peace with any negative thoughts that may be blocking you from your heart's deepest desires.

If you want to know what you are thinking, examine your feelings. Really get in touch with them. Your feelings never lie. They tell you if you are connected to who you really are in the moment or not.

Of course, you mustn't forget your spoken words, as they have tremendous power, especially when directed inward. Whether positive or negative, they have the power to help or hinder your quest for a healthier you. In Missing Peace #9: Choose Carefully the Words Following "I Am," you are given guidance on how to change the station from statements of negative self-talk to those evoking better feelings and thoughts.

Missing Peace #8: What You Think about, You Bring About

> All that we are is a result of what we have thought.
> —The Buddha

What you think about, you bring about. Really?

If someone told me this five years ago, I would've listened politely, laughed quietly to myself, and then dismissed the idea as nothing more than new age baloney. *I live in the real world of things, and if I can't see it, I don't believe it,* I would've thought. I mean, if I can't physically see a thought, how is it possible that it can manifest into something physical? It doesn't make logical sense.

As I mentally scan through my life up until this point, there is no doubt in my mind that this Missing Peace is indeed true. It's funny how circumstances align just right in life to teach you the lessons you have to learn in order to become the person you were meant to be.

For example, about ten years ago, I was standing in the checkout line at my local office supply store. Because it was the New Year, an assortment of daily tear-off calendars was on display near the checkout line. One calendar in particular caught my eye; it was called "The Secret." The title intrigued me, so I decided to add it to my shopping basket.

From the cover, I expected to see a series of daily motivational quotes; however, that wasn't the case. I quickly became disappointed as the days went by, tearing page after page, hoping for some inspiration to pop out at me. Not only were there no famous quotes or pieces of ancient wisdom to glean, as each day passed, I became more and more confused by the calendar's message: paragraphs and paragraphs about your thoughts. I simply didn't get it.

Fast-forward five years. I was having lunch with a very dear friend of mine named Jeff. He's one of my favorite people in the world, an extremely intuitive gentleman who knows all the right questions to ask in order to get you thinking.

As we were waiting for our lunch to be served, I shared with Jeff that earlier that day, I received a phone call from a company in another part of the country that was looking for a dietitian to offer telephonic counseling services to their clients. I remarked at how strange and coincidental it was because I had been searching for an additional revenue stream to fund my growing business.

Jeff looked at me, chuckled nonchalantly, and asked, "You mean you don't know how that happened, Melanie?"

Perplexed at his question and sort of annoyed by what I perceived to be a sarcastic response, I answered as honestly as I could, "No. How?"

"Don't you realize that you made that happen?" he replied.

Smiling his big, warm, and handsome smile, Jeff went on to talk about our thoughts being energy and having the ability to reach out and influence others, even in different parts of the world. I was intrigued on the one hand, but on the other, I thought he was half-nuts. We went on to have a beautiful lunch together, and then I left the conversation there.

Later that week, it hit me. Was Jeff talking about the Secret? It sounded familiar; perhaps that's why I wasn't fully buying it. Remember, I read about this stuff for 365 days and was quite soured by it. Again, I didn't get it at the time. At that moment, I connected two dots and let it go.

Over the course of several years, a series of events, circumstances, and chance meetings led me to the works of spiritual teachers like the Buddha and authors such as Abraham Hicks, Wayne Dyer, Deepak Chopra, Napoleon Hill, Joseph Benner, and Neville Goddard, all individuals who speak to some degree about the law of attraction and living in the present moment. It's often said that when the student is ready, the teacher will appear, and boy, was I ready.

My entire world seemed to change right before my eyes, and all of a sudden, everything I thought I understood about life was turned on its side. I began to question everything. I started connecting dot after dot after dot, and a tremendous amount of clarity washed over me. The veil was lifted.

As Steve Jobs once said:

You can't connect the dots looking forward, you can only connect them looking backward. So you have to trust that the dots will somehow connect in your future. You have to trust in something—your gut, destiny, life, karma, whatever. This approach has never let me down, and it has made all the difference in my life.[6]

I began to realize that the painful experience I went through with binge eating disorder was not only brought about by my thoughts; it was a dot that had to happen in order for me to move forward and live the life of my dreams. Yes, I believe beyond a shadow of a doubt that I attracted binge eating disorder into my life.

Another way to speak of this phenomenon called the law of attraction is, what you focus on, expands. Focusing on undesirable states that offer a great deal of inner contrast, such as lack, poverty, obesity, and disease, will draw more of these things into your life.

Since thoughts are energy and, literally, things, you want to be extra careful not to feed anything to your mind that you don't want to come to life. I suggest very strongly that you clean up the thoughts you think about yourself and the contrasting experiences in your life. Pretend that every thought you have will come to life.

---

[6] Stanford University. "Text of Steve Jobs' Commencement Address (2005)." *Stanford News*, June 12, 2017.

At first glance, the word *contrast* might conjure up negative feelings, but it's not necessarily a negative thing. In fact, it can be quite helpful as a tool. I define *contrast* as an experience or situation that helps clarify what you really want. It can occur in any of these areas of your life: health, body shape, fitness level, food, relationships, finances, career, and spirituality.

Jalaluddin Rumi, a thirteenth-century Sufi mystic and poet, offers a unique way of appreciating all the thoughts and emotions we experience as human beings. Rather than deny them, he asks you to invite them in, with gratitude in your heart.

The Guest House[7]

This being human is a guest house.
Every morning a new arrival.

A joy, a depression, a meanness,
some momentary awareness comes
As an unexpected visitor.

Welcome and entertain them all!
Even if they're a crowd of sorrows,
who violently sweep your house
empty of its furniture,
still treat each guest honorably.
He may be clearing you out
for some new delight.

---

[7] "The Guest House by Mewlana Jalaluddin Rumi," from *Mewlana Jalaluddin Rumi: Famous Poems, Famous Poets.*

The dark thought, the shame, the malice,
meet them at the door laughing,
and invite them in.

Be grateful for whoever comes,
because each has been sent
as a guide from beyond.

For example, let's say you are out of shape and therefore experiencing contrast in your level of physical fitness. This contrast helps you identify what you *do* want: a fit and healthy body. So if you don't wish to occupy an out-of-shape body, stop talking about your unfit body and calling attention to it. Instead, acknowledge and welcome the contrast, and then focus on what you desire instead.

During my journey with binge eating disorder, all I thought about was losing weight and how unhappy I was with my current body. This unhappiness multiplied, and Divine energy gave me more of what I was giving my attention to. I got to the point where I was drowning in a tangled web of food and emotions. I couldn't take it anymore. I had enough of the binging and overexercising, feeling guilty about food, inability to sense fullness, and total detachment from the true essence of me. This was the most contrast I ever experienced in my life, and it helped me to identify what I *did* want: a life free of food addiction and obsession. I wanted to be able to sit down to a delicious dinner at a nice restaurant with Wayne and not focus so much on the food. I wanted to enjoy the company and environment, and then walk away from the table without thinking about my next meal. I felt this deep within my soul. I felt, even if just for a few moments, what it would feel like to be free.

Here's what the entire process looks like:

> Make peace with, embrace, and appreciate what *is* (your body as it now is). Decide what you want (a fit and healthy body), and put that desire in your mind without calling repeated attention to what *is* (your body as it now is). Imagine what it will feel like to occupy this fit and healthy body. How will it feel in your clothes? See yourself in the mirror staring back. See it as already done. Believe that you occupy a fit and healthy body, and release resistance to any thought or feeling to the contrary, such as *Yeah, but I've tried to improve my body in the past by dieting and spending countless hours in the gym, with no results.*

> Now it's time to take action. This piece must not be forgotten. A fit and healthy body isn't magically created by thought alone—you must take action. Eat more Earthfoods, move your body more, and offer it gratitude for keeping you alive all these years. Do this all while releasing attachment to the outcome. Let go, and watch your body as it changes.

Divine energy will bring you exactly what you place your attention upon, whether you want it or not. So if you aren't satisfied with your body as it is today, for Pete's sake, stop focusing on it, get to thinking about the healthy body of your dreams, and take action; it will become a reality.

More on Taking Action

If you're experiencing contrast in any area of your life and want it to change, it's essential that you do something about it.

It's easy to sit and complain, but if you aren't taking consistent and persistent action to change an undesirable situation, you really have no business bellyaching in the first place. And trust me, your friends and family don't want to listen to it, either.

Do something, anything, to move the needle in a more positive direction. For example, if you're experiencing a health contrast that you wish was different, such as diabetes, you can choose to take action and exchange all your sugar-sweetened beverages for water.

If you're out of shape and can't climb a flight of stairs without huffing and puffing, you can choose to take action and commit to walking at a brisk pace for thirty minutes each day to strengthen your cardiovascular system.

The Power of Your Beliefs

Your belief system plays a big role, especially when it comes to the state of your health. Dr. Bruce Lipton, the author of *The Biology of Belief*, speaks of something called epigenetics. In a blog post from July 15, 2014, Lipton defined epigenetics this way:

Instead of the widely held, largely deterministic belief among biologists about genetics, namely that our genes "control" or "determine" us, it is rather the case that our genes respond to cues in their environment, such as one's experience and perception of, or beliefs regarding your own life.

Dr. Lipton went on to explain the science behind epigenetics in an August 28, 2014 blog post:

In a plastic tissue culture dish, the composition of the growth medium (environment) controls the fate of the cells. The human body is, by definition, a "skin-covered culture dish" containing ~50,000,000,000,000 (fifty trillion) cells. The cells are maintained by a culture medium ... popularly known as blood. The chemical composition of the blood is the equivalent of the culture medium used in the plastic culture dishes. Changing the composition of the blood's chemistry is the same as changing a culture's growth medium. The brain is the regulatory organ that regulates and maintains the chemical composition of the blood. The brain's control of the blood's chemistry is linked to our perceptions (mind) and emotions (reflecting chemical signals in the blood). When you have a perception of love, the brain releases oxytocin (love hormone that regulates the body's metabolism and supports growth), serotonin and growth hormone, ALL chemicals that when added to cells in a culture dish will enhance growth and health of the cells. In contrast when a person is in fear, their brain releases stress hormones (cortisol, norepinephrine and histamine) that shut down a cell's growth processes and inhibits the immune system, which happens to be completely unsustainable for life.

He ends by stating the following:

> Your thoughts adjust the brain's control of the blood, which in turn controls that fate of the cells … MIND OVER BODY!

I invite you to read the above paragraph again so that you can fully understand the power of your thoughts and beliefs in all areas of your life. Essentially, Dr. Lipton is suggesting that your mind controls your genes.

You are not a victim of your genetics. You can change your mind any way you desire, positive or negative. A victim mentality of "High cholesterol runs in my family, therefore I am doomed to get high cholesterol" can very easily be changed to the empowerment mentality of "I am in complete control of my health, and I call the shots. I am healthy and well, and my blood is clean and pure."

It really is a matter of choice. Choose to think and believe in an empowering manner; what can it hurt?

Still, you may not be convinced that thoughts become things and have the power to affect your physical world. Let's move to an example offering evidence you can see with your own two eyes.

Dr. Masaru Emoto, a Japanese author, photographer, and researcher, did some mind-blowing work on how thoughts and feelings affect physical reality.

Using samples of newly formed ice crystals, Dr. Emoto showed how their patterns changed shape and color depending on the nature of the words, concentrated thoughts, and music they were exposed to. For example, when exposed to kind and loving words, such as "gratitude," "love," and "peace," the water crystals formed beautifully colored snowflake patterns. Interestingly, when exposed to negative statement, like "You're a fool," "You disgust me," and "You're evil," the crystals formed asymmetrical patterns with dull colors.

This research opens up an entire new world of possibilities on how the power of your thoughts creates your reality. Just imagine the state of health you can create for yourself by simply shifting your thoughts and beliefs just a little bit. You have so much more control than you think.

This Shouldn't Feel Like Work

There is a noticeable difference between my earlier years of manifestation compared to my most recent, however. Once I discovered the notion that thoughts become things, I put way too much effort into the process. I was attached to the outcome, which caused me to search for the hows, namely, "How will I make this happen?" I was clinging so tightly to the outcome that I almost let my entire world revolve around what I was attempting to make come true in my life. It felt too much like work.

One afternoon while exercising on the elliptical machine, I decided to tune into a Buddhist podcast to pass the time. The topic of discussion was "clinging," which is one of the causes of suffering in our life. The instructor explained clinging by comparing it to rope burn. He asked us to grab a nearby object, so I chose a pencil and continued to listen for his instruction, feeling increasingly intrigued. He told us to hold the object as tight as we could with all of our strength, and he would tell us when to let go. As I held on to the pencil, squeezing as hard as I could, my hand started to burn and feel weak. After about twenty seconds, he asked us to let go of the object, and I did. I instantly felt relief.

So what was the point of this exercise? When you cling to something so tightly, whether it's a pencil or an outcome, person, situation, or job, there's a lot of energy and effort involved. It becomes exhausting, even painful. The instant you surrender and let go of the situation, you feel immediate relief.

His message really resonated with me because about a week earlier, I had to make the heartbreaking decision to put my seventeen-year-old cat to sleep due to an illness. If you've ever had to make this decision, you know how emotionally difficult it can be. I was devastated and, quite honestly, didn't know how to handle the flood of emotions I was experiencing. I'd never been through the dreaded experience of letting go of a pet this close to me; I couldn't bear the raw pain I was feeling. It was like an exposed nerve that kept getting plucked by my emotions.

During the rope burn exercise, I envisioned the squeezing of the pencil as my emotions and attachment to the pain. When I let go, I envisioned myself letting go of Molly, my beloved feline friend, who gave me so much unconditional love and friendship all of those seventeen years. From that moment on, things were different. I still had a bit of emotional pain, but I was no longer clinging to her.

How does all of this relate to your thoughts becoming things? Nothing about this process should feel like work. If you desire something, believe and behave as if it is already yours, feel what it will feel like when it's yours, release attachment, and let go. This is where the magic happens.

I believe that the act of clinging and attachment blocks your desires from being fulfilled. If it feels like emotional effort and dis-ease in my body, this is my indication that something isn't right, that a blockage is occurring. In every case, as soon as I detach from the outcome, feelings of ease wash over my body. This is my internal indication that I've cleared the block and am in a state of allowing.

Ask and Allow: Five Steps to Manifest Anything in Your Life

Author and teacher Abraham Hicks explains this process beautifully by offering the following five steps to manifesting anything in your life:[8]

Step 1: Ask for what you want. Contrast causes you as a human being to do this.

For me, the asking came in the form of a strong desire for a peaceful relationship with food and my body.

Step 2: Source, Universe, God, or whatever you call it, answers.

I believe our desires are always answered, but because we focus our attention so heavily on the contrast and attach so strongly to the outcome, we block our desires from manifesting.

Step 3: Get in the receptive mode, where you allow yourself to receive.

This step is of particular importance because according to Abraham, it's when you recognize that the way you feel is your indication of whether you're allowing yourself to receive or not. When you feel good, you're in

---

[8] Esther and Jerry Hicks, *Ask and It Is Given: Learning to Manifest Your Desires.* Hay House Publications, 2004.

the state of allowing; when you feel not-so-good, you're cutting yourself off from allowing. Positive emotion can feel like any of the following: joy, bliss, clarity, abundance, happiness, laughter, peace, gratitude, hope, inspiration, and love.

Step 4: You own your desire and practice it. Here, you care about the way you feel, and it is so important to you that you feel good that you won't allow anything to stand in your way of achieving good feeling thoughts.

Make it your number one priority, let go, and focus on feeling amazing.

Step 5: You stop beating up on yourself and welcome contrast. When it happens, you acknowledge its value for the clarity it will bring.

A simple example is when I get stuck behind someone who is driving under the speed limit. For some reason, this petty source of contrast really frustrates me. Negative, bad-feeling thoughts and words race out of my mind and mouth: *Why can't they speed up? For Pete's sake, you can at least go the speed limit.* Thanks to the teachings of Abraham, I have found a way to turn this contrasting experience around to work in my favor. Now, when I get stuck behind a slowpoke driver, I first pretend this person is my mother or grandmother. Would I react this way? Of course not. Then, I conclude that there must be a reason why I'm being forced to slow down. Is this person helping me avoid a collision on the freeway?

I can't lie: I still get frustrated driving behind these people, but now I am able to quickly pull myself out of the negative downward spiral. Then I turn up the classical music, put my car in cruise control, and coast at a nice and steady 30 miles per hour.

Thanks to the teachings of Abraham Hicks and others, I can now say that when I experience contrast in any area of my life, whether it's in the form of a slow driver, a disagreeable person, a traffic jam, or an unexpected roadblock on my path, I first appreciate it and then focus on what I want instead of lack. Finally, I get in a better feeling place and do whatever it takes to get me there. I like to call it Operation Mood-Booster.

Meditation, listening to classical music, writing in my gratitude journal, taking a walk in nature, petting my cat, hugging my husband, or taking a few long, slow, focused deep breaths are all mood-boosters I have in my arsenal, ready to activate at any given moment. Most of all, I release resistance and stop trying to make it happen. Sure, I take action, but inside, there is a quiet knowing that my desire is already fulfilled. I don't worry about how it will happen because I have undying faith that it will.

Make Peace Exercise: Bring about Your Desires

1. Pay attention to your dominant thoughts, and write the first thought that comes to your mind in each the following areas of your life:
   a. health
   b. body
   c. family relationships
   d. romantic relationship
   e. financial situation
   f. career
   g. spirituality

2. Make peace with any negative thoughts and feelings you have about the above areas of your life. Accept and surrender to what is. Next, declare below what it is you would like to manifest in each of these areas:
   a. health
   b. body
   c. family relationships
   d. romantic relationship
   e. financial situation
   f. career
   g. spirituality

3. List one action step you can take today toward the manifestation of your desires in each of these core areas of your life:
   a. health

b. body
c. family relationships
d. romantic relationship
e. financial situation
f. career
g. spirituality

4. Release attachment and clinging to any outcome, and instead, pay very careful attention to your feelings. Remember, when you experience a positive emotion, this is your cue that you are in a state of allowing your desires to manifest. When negative emotions surface in any of these areas, immediately put into action a mood-boosting thought, affirmation, or action that you can draw upon to elevate you so you feel slightly better. Make a list of five mood-boosters below:
    a. Mood-booster #1: _____
    b. Mood-booster #2: _____
    c. Mood-booster #3: _____
    d. Mood-booster #4: _____
    e. Mood-booster #5: _____

Return to Your Light of Peace

Shine a light on your thoughts. As you take in a long, slow, deep breath, feel your Light of Peace radiate throughout your entire body. As a thought floats into your field of awareness, simply notice it. How does the thought make you feel? Uneasy, anxious, and contracted? Or peaceful, happy, and expanded? If necessary, allow your Light of Peace to guide you toward a slightly improved thought, one that evokes a more positive emotional state.

Recommended Peace of Health Shake

Strawberry Lemon Surprise Shake

7 Earthfood Servings ♥♥♥♥♥♥♥

12–16 oz. unsweetened almond, cashew, coconut, or flax milk
2 tbsp. Earthfood Powder
¼ of a small avocado, peeled and seeded
1 cup fresh organic kale
1 cup shredded red cabbage
1 tbsp. fresh ginger
¼ of a lemon, with rind
½ cup frozen cauliflower (surprise)
½ cup frozen organic strawberries

Instructions:

Add all ingredients to a high-powered blender (such as Vitamix, Blendtec, or Ninja) in the order listed and blend until smooth.

Nutrition Facts: Calories: 320; Total Fat: 20 g; Saturated Fat: 8 g; Sodium: 200 mg; Potassium: 680 mg; Total Carbohydrates: 31 g; Dietary Fiber: 14 g; Net Carbohydrates: 17 g; Sugar: 8 g (no added sugar); Protein: 13 g

Note: Peace of Health shakes are not sweet, and that is by design. Sweetness is a trained preference, one that can be changed. The goal is to recalibrate your taste buds so that you begin to pick up the natural sweetness of the small amount of fruit in the shakes, without having to add sweetener or extra fruit. For a sweeter shake, refer to the tips offered in the "Do-It-Yourself Shakes" section at the beginning of the book.

Missing Peace #9: Choose Carefully the Words Following "I Am"

> I will not let anyone walk through my
> mind with their dirty feet.
> —Mahatma Gandhi

Perhaps you don't say it out loud, but have you ever caught yourself thinking things like, *I am so stupid, I am so hopeless,* or *I am so fat*? Sure, we all do. I remember not long ago, I was putting groceries away, and instead of putting the eggs in the refrigerator, I put them in the pantry. "I am so stupid," I exclaimed. Those words just rolled off my tongue without a second thought. This is a common problem, and we don't even realize we're saying it. We are conditioned to respond this way. We may have heard our mother say, "I am so fat," when she looked at herself in the mirror, and we just grew up thinking that's what you say when you're unhappy with your appearance.

Words have tremendous power, especially when directed inward. Whether positive or negative, they have the power

123

to help or hinder your quest for a healthier you, especially when feelings are attached to those words.

I'm not suggesting that you deny your thoughts and feelings, because that would be like sweeping them under the rug. Understand, the not-so-good feeling thoughts have their place too, because without them, you would fail to learn, grow, and strive for more. Acknowledge them and the feelings they evoke. Respect them as a piece of your humanness, and then move to a better feeling thought, one that will spark a kinder, gentler "I am" statement.

For example, just the other day, I caught myself saying, "I am so tired," and while this was true (I was physically and emotionally drained), the second those words escaped my lips, I felt even more drained. What could I have said to lighten the effects? Sometimes, saying nothing is the most appropriate response, but we often like to hear ourselves talk. If this is the case, and you just have to say something or you'll burst, how about something like, "My body and mind feel tired; what I really need is to take five minutes to myself and relax," or even more powerful, "I have just enough energy to complete the task at hand; in fact, I feel good! But afterward, I'm going to settle down for some me time."

I want you to pretend that everything you say will turn into an instant manifestation. So, if you exclaim, "I am so fat," pretend fifty extra pounds will immediately appear on your body. After all, it's Divine energy giving you what you are placing your attention on, whether it's wanted or not.

The following tool will confirm the tremendous power of your words: Make a list of the negative comments you make to yourself, and then imagine yourself saying them to a beloved friend or family member; your mom, for example. Would you ever say the following to your mother: "Mom, you are so fat," or "Mom, you are so lazy and disgusting"? Of course, you wouldn't; that would be hurtful. And besides, you love your mother and just don't say things like that to people you love. So why then do we find it perfectly acceptable to say these words to ourselves?

Understand that if you say something negative, you are thinking it. And if you are thinking it, you are most certainly experiencing inner feelings of lack, shame, discontent, defeat, sadness, anxiety, depression, guilt, helplessness, and unworthiness. You feel downright awful. That is no way to go through this amazing ride called life. When you feel any negative emotion, it's a clear sign that you are creating a disconnect between you and your higher self.

You have an obligation to feel good. Feeling positive emotion is a true indicator that you allow your Light of Peace to shine. Doesn't it stand to reason, then, that if you want to feel good and connected, you should start with your thoughts? If you want to feel better, just reach for a better feeling thought. It's that simple. And of course, the better you feel, the better your life will become: more happiness, healthier choices, better relationships, and the list of goodness goes on.

In spite of what you may think, you have complete control over your thoughts. For example, you can choose to look at your aching knee and think, *I am so old; aging sure is a bitch*, or you can think, *I am as young as I allow myself to feel. Sure, I may have overdone it yesterday during my workout at the gym, so next time, I'll be sure to stretch afterward. In fact, I'd better stretch right now.*

Another example: Instead of thinking of yourself as fat and hopeless, shift to a better feeling thought: *I am voluptuous and full of promise.* Which one makes you feel better? Also, with improved feelings come better choices. If you are making food choices from a mind-set of *I am fat,* the majority of the foods that you buy and eat will be unhealthy comfort foods that do not serve you. What I'm offering you is not a form of denial; it's simply choosing to look at the situation with more light than darkness.

Many unpleasant thoughts about yourself are a result of other people's opinions and expectations, and your perception of their opinions and expectations. Make no mistake: your opinion is the only one that matters.

One of my favorite quotes is by Jack Canfield, author of the famous *Chicken Soup for the Soul* books. He says, "What others think about you is none of your business." I think that's brilliant. I keep it at the forefront of my mind whenever I'm tempted to give a damn about what others think of me, and then I take myself through the following mental exercise:

> I imagine myself in a room with that person, and as they give their opinion, I decide if it's helpful or not. If it is, I take it into consideration and allow it to stay in the room. If it's negative or not helpful, I open a nearby

window and watch their words as they float outside, out of my space. Then I close the window. No harm done.

Never let anyone influence the words that follow your "I am."

You have the power to change the station when what is being played on the current one makes you feel anything less than peaceful. When negative emotions arise, tempting you to blurt out unkind words about yourself, acknowledge and release them. Turn the station, open the window, and let them go. Then reach for the best feeling thoughts you can, declare a positive "I am" statement, and watch what happens. You'll be amazed at how good you feel and even more amazed that you and you alone were responsible.

Words have tremendous power. Use them wisely, especially when those words follow "I am."

Make Peace Exercise: Shine a Light on Your "I Am" Statements

1. For one week, carry a small notebook with you wherever you go, and listen for your "I am" statements. Whether you say them out loud or think them in your mind, write them in your notebook, leaving a blank line after each statement.

2. At the end of each day, review your list of "I am" statements, but do not judge them. Instead, write a better feeling statement on the blank line below any negative statements. Read your new "I am"

statement out loud at least three times, and pay attention to how it makes you feel.

Return to Your Light of Peace

Your Light of Peace represents unconditional love. Take a couple of conscious breaths to bring yourself into the present moment, and join with your Light of Peace. Ask the question, Who am I? Listen for and feel the answer.

Recommended Peace of Health Shake

Melanie's Go-To Power Shake

8 Earthfood Servings ♥♥♥♥♥♥♥♥

12 oz. unsweetened almond, cashew, coconut, or flax milk
1 tsp. maca powder
2 tbsp. Earthfood Powder
¼ lemon with rind
1 tbsp. fresh ginger
1 tbsp. fresh turmeric
½ of a small avocado, peeled and seeded
2 cups fresh organic kale
½ cup frozen wild blueberries

Instructions:

Add all ingredients to a high-powered blender (such as Vitamix, Blendtec, or Ninja) in the order listed and blend until smooth.

Nutrition Facts: Calories: 400; Total Fat: 29 g; Saturated Fat: 9 g; Sodium: 195 mg; Potassium: 685 mg; Total Carbohydrates: 40 g; Dietary Fiber: 16 g; Net Carbohydrates: 24 g; Sugar: 8 g (no added sugar); Protein: 14 g

Note: Peace of Health shakes are not sweet, and that is by design. Sweetness is a trained preference, one that can be changed. The goal is to recalibrate your taste buds so that you begin to pick up the natural sweetness of the small amount of fruit in the shakes, without having to add sweetener or extra fruit. For a sweeter shake, refer to the tips offered in the "Do-It-Yourself Shakes" section at the beginning of the book.

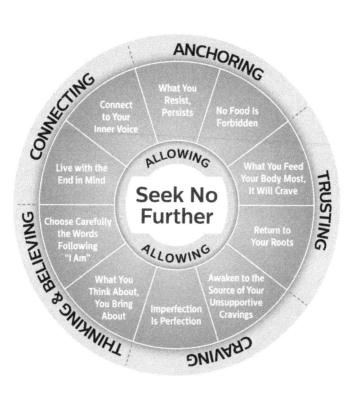

Chapter 6: Connecting

Missing Peace #10: Live with the End in Mind
Missing Peace #11: Connect to Your Inner Voice

Next, you experience the Connecting phase, that is, making space to connect to who you really are.

In Missing Peace #10: Live with the End in Mind, you are introduced to a visualization tool called the End in Mind meditation, where you are guided to see yourself in the body of your dreams. From there, you learn how to embody that person, making the choices they would make, while believing and feeling that you already are that person. It is quite a magical experience.

In Missing Peace #11: Connect to Your Inner Voice, you learn how to tap into the voice of your higher self, the self that only knows health and peace. To do this, you must get quiet, tune in, and trust your silent, knowing observer. Meditation, which involves quieting your mind and focusing on your breath, is the most effective way to bring yourself into the present moment, where all of your power rests. When you connect to your inner voice, really settle in and listen, making healthy choices is incredibly effortless.

Missing Peace #10: Live with the End in Mind

First say to yourself what you would be;
and then do what you have to do.
—Epictetus

When I ask my clients and audiences why they feel it's so difficult to change their current lifestyle habits, I usually get answers like "It's too time consuming" or "I miss my favorite foods." While these are legitimate, supporting reasons for falling off track, they are not at the core of why we really fail to sustain healthy change.

The real reason we fail is because we continue to make choices as the version of ourselves we are trying to change, the one offering contrast, with high cholesterol and fifty extra pounds to lose. We act as the one who, in the past, chased after good health by seeking it outside of ourselves, in the next diet or exercise program. We aren't living and making choices as if we already are the picture of perfect health.

In order to change this, we must first change how we see ourselves. In fact, how you treat your body, including what you feed it and whether you exercise or not, is directly related to how you see your body.

If you see your body as fat, unhealthy, gross, or broken, that is exactly how you will treat it. On the other hand, if you see it as a healthy temple, a five-star resort, you will treat it as such.

When I'm approached by someone seeking to lose weight, and they say, "I am so fat and out of shape. I need to lose fifty pounds," it's no wonder they haven't lost any weight or have been unable to maintain a weight loss. They see their body as fat and out of shape, and that's how they habitually treat it. I can almost guarantee they will never reach their goal; not with that attitude.

Understand that if you remain stuck in what I call "what-is land" and refuse to see yourself as anything *but* someone who is diabetic, overweight, or whatever your current ailments are, you'll never be able to make the necessary changes to create this higher vision of yourself—you as a healthy temple, a five-star resort, and so on. You must already see yourself as the temple. You must begin with the desired end in mind and *live* from that end.

How Do You See Yourself?

If you always seem to struggle with creating lasting, healthy change, I'd like you to try this exercise:

Look at yourself in the mirror, directly into the eyes staring back at you. What do you see? Who do you see? A tired, worn-out person who is addicted to sugar and processed food? Or a vibrant, healthy individual in love with life, one who makes healthy choices because it makes her feel good? Someone who respects herself and knows she only makes choices to serve her higher self? If you see the former, or any version of the former, that is exactly what you will receive. If, on the other hand, you see that vibrant woman staring back, you will get those results. You become what you think about, so why not think of and see yourself as the product of your desire already manifested?

Today, right this very moment, you are the sum total of all of your past thoughts. So if you aren't happy with what you've been getting, start putting the good stuff in, and make a firm commitment to live from that end. See yourself in the body of your dreams. What does it look and feel like? Once you can see that picture as clear and detailed as your favorite piece of art, it's time to embody that person and begin making the choices they would make. Even though you may love them, a healthy and vibrant individual would not eat doughnuts for breakfast. It just wouldn't make sense.

This isn't a matter of exercising willpower but rather an almost unconscious practice of living with the desired end in mind.

Once you get this down, it's very important that you believe and feel, with everything you are, that you are *already* this person. The beauty of this is, the more often you drink the smoothie for breakfast instead of the sugar-laden, overpriced coffee drink with a blueberry muffin on the side, the more your body will crave that smoothie. Remember Missing Peace #4: What You Feed Your Body Most, It Will Crave?

End in Mind Meditation

The following is a visualization tool that I've developed to help you practice this Missing Peace and live as the end product of your desires.

Sit in a comfortable position, either on the floor on a meditation cushion or in a chair. Maintain a nice tall posture, and close your eyes. Begin breathing normally, paying specific attention to the air as it flows through your nostrils and into your lungs on the inhale, and as it moves out of your lungs and nostrils on the exhale.

Picture a beautiful blue mist, representing the clean, pure air that you breathe. Watch it as it flows in as you take a breath. As you exhale, observe the air as it flows out of your nostrils, only this time, the air is black in color. Inhale pure, clean, healthy thoughts and energy (blue mist), and exhale impurities, stale energy, negative thoughts, and ill-health (black mist).

When thoughts enter your field of awareness, gently acknowledge them and then escort them out of your mind. It helps to imagine these thoughts as if they are sitting on top of beautifully colored leaves in a downward stream. Watch each thought as it is being carried away by the current. Right now, you have no worries. Not a care in the world. You are in a state of infinite possibilities.

As you continue to pay attention to the beautiful blue mist of pure, clean air flowing into your lungs and the black mist as it exits your body, think of an area of your current state of health that you are seeking to change. It could be a food addiction or your blood pressure, body shape, blood sugar, cholesterol, or a specific disease that is currently living in your body. Embrace this situation with love and kindness, and see it in front of you as if it were a separate entity from your physical body. Speak to it. Tell it you appreciate it being part of your life to teach you the lessons that you needed to learn. Express genuine gratitude for it, and then graciously request that it leave your body, your temple. While still focusing on your breath, watch as the condition or situation exits your body, being escorted by the black mist.

Feel into your new body, the temple that now lacks the past condition. See a beautiful sunrise as it makes its appearance in your cells and shines new healing light upon every tissue, vessel, and organ. Feel what it feels like to own this new body, the energy, freedom, and vibrancy you now possess. Continue breathing and focusing on how your body feels in its new skin. As you admire this amazing creation, visualize yourself making a clean, healthy choice at your next meal. Feel the energy as the food you eat begins to break down and flow through your bloodstream, infusing every cell with life, love, and energy, knowing that you were responsible for nourishing your temple with pure goodness.

I can't emphasize enough the importance of living as the end product of your desire and making choices from this place, as this person. Understand that you are this person. Believe and feel yourself inhabiting this new you. Feel the energy as it courses through your veins. Take a good look in the mirror, and see the new you. The beauty of this visualization meditation is that it allows you to create any picture of yourself that you desire. There are no rules.

Embodying the New You: Five Thoughts to Consider

Here are five thoughts to consider as you go about your journey, creating this expanded version of yourself:

1. Focus on how you want to feel.

Upon deciding what (and how much) to eat, focus on the feeling of the end result by asking yourself, "How do I want to feel after this meal?" This very question is at the core of living a healthy life. By describing the feeling, such as satisfied, energized, in control, proud, healthy, or light, this question forces you to place yourself at the receiving end of your decision.

2. Only you know what is best for you.

You must make sure that the picture you paint of your highest and healthiest self is something you (and only you) desire. It doesn't matter what other people think or what they believe is best for you. As Steve Jobs said so eloquently in his 2005 Stanford University commencement address:

Your time is limited, so don't waste it living someone else's life. Don't be trapped by dogma—which is living with the results of other people's thinking. Don't let the noise of others' opinions drown out your own inner voice. And most important, have the courage to follow your heart and intuition. They somehow already know what you truly want. Everything else is secondary.

3. Ignore past failed attempts.

Never allow past failed attempts to muddy your ultimate vision of yourself. Those attempts came from old thoughts, and they are no longer you. Right this very moment, you are setting the stage for the new you, and your dominant thoughts from here on out will mold who you are to become. Imagine big.

4. Anticipate resistance and make it work *for* you.

In 2015, therapist and best-selling author Marisa Peer shared a brilliant take on the power of your mind at an annual event called Awesomeness Fest. She stated, "Your brain does what it thinks you want." How I interpret this is, if you want to do something, but have built up resistance to it, like exercising or meal planning, it is perfectly acceptable to trick your mind into believing it is a joyful experience. I use this idea on a daily basis to help me push through resistance and live with the end in mind.

Not long ago, I was warming up on the treadmill at the gym. Even though I visualized myself at the end of my workout, feeling energized and on top of the world, as I looked behind me at the rows of free weights, I felt a wave of resistance wash over me. Traditionally, I've always preferred cardiovascular activity to resistance training, but I do both because they are both important for a strong body.

On this particular day, I was really dreading my weight routine, to the point I started feeling cranky and resentful. As I neared the end of my run, I could feel the resistance continue to build. *Ugh,* I thought. *I really, really, really don't want to do weights today. I'd rather just go home. Besides, I am feeling extra tired and hungry. Maybe I'll just skip it this time.*

As I took a step back and watched my mind go down the familiar road of endless excuses—the excuses I hear from people on almost a daily basis for why they skipped their workout—I thought to myself, *Melanie, you can turn this around. Instead of complaining, why not flip the switch and get excited about your weight routine? Why not choose to feel excitement instead of dread? After all, it is your choice. Go ahead and trick your mind.*

So I did just that. I flipped the switch. I turned around and looked at the weights, the very same weights I was cursing just moments before, and I said to myself, *I can't wait to wrap up this cardio session and hit the weights. I love how I feel when I'm done: the strength and balance, the good muscle soreness that wakes up my body and strengthens my bones with each repetition.* I counted down the seconds as the treadmill slowed to a stop, anticipating with eager excitement the good that I was about to do my body. I felt like I was seeing through a totally new pair of eyes. Guess what? It worked. I had the most amazing workout of my life. Even though I didn't physically do anything different to create such a stellar workout, I flipped the switch on my attitude and imagined myself at the end of it, and it made all the difference in the world.

One thing I know for sure is that it's really easy to talk yourself out of a task you see as dreaded or to choose one food over another, even though the other is clearly better for you.

Your mind moves so fast that in the blink of an eye, you blurt out, "Lasagna with French bread, please," instead of the grilled salmon with broccoli. It took a split-second for you to settle on lasagna because, well, it's lasagna, and no one in their right mind would willingly choose salmon over layers of cheesy lasagna bathing in zesty marinara sauce. Because of the lightning-speed nature of your mind, it is more important than ever that you develop the skill of making choices with your desired end in mind.

5. Be consistent.

If your goal is to physically become the person of your dreams, it is your duty to be consistent in your new way of thinking and behaving. An easy way to do this is to make a commitment to practice the EIM visualization meditation first thing every morning until it becomes part of you, until you effortlessly make choices from that place.

I invite you to take this day-by-day and meal-by-meal. Instead of thinking, *I am now the perfect weight with perfect health and must never eat another potato chip as long as I live*, relax into your food choices. Remember Missing Peace #2: What You Resist, Persists, and Missing Peace #3: No Food Is Forbidden. Saying that you will never allow a potato chip to touch your lips is a declaration destined for disaster.

Instead, on day one of the new you, think to yourself, *I am now the perfect weight with perfect health. What does the new me want for breakfast? What will nourish me and keep me as healthy and vibrant as I look and feel today?* Then make your choice. For example, the answer that comes to you may very well be a spinach, blueberry, and avocado smoothie. After you nourish your body with the smoothie and feel amazing, plan an equally nourishing lunch to keep the positive momentum going.

When faced with a situation that the old you would've given into—such as helping yourself to a doughnut in the break room—you now approach the situation like this: *I am so healthy and feel so amazing. Although that glazed doughnut looks and smells amazing, and I have full permission to eat it, I am going to pass because I know it will drain me of the energy and vitality that I've built up so far.* From there, you move on to your next meal or snack.

Do you see how this works? Live moment to moment as the new you already manifested, and before you know it, you will begin to crave this new way of thinking and behaving with the end in mind.

Make Peace Exercise: Live with Your End Desire in Mind

Spend three to five minutes every morning practicing your EIM visualization meditation. You may use the version I offered earlier or create one that feels right for you. The key is to see yourself as the product of your desire already manifested. Believe and feel, with everything you are, that you are already this person. Because you are.

Return to Your Light of Peace

By suggesting you live with the end in mind, it may seem like I am asking you to go into the future, therefore taking you out of the present moment. This is not so.

To live can only happen right here and now, in this present moment, in this breath. To live with the end in mind simply means you are drawing that higher, healthier version of yourself toward you, stepping into her shoes, and making choices as if you already are that which you desire to be. Because you are.

So get present. Breathe into your Light of Peace, your higher self, the one who already knows what you truly want and is waiting to deliver this highest physical version of you, to you. All you have to do is allow.

Recommended Peace of Health Shake

Peachy Keen Shake

7 Earthfood Servings ♥ ♥ ♥ ♥ ♥ ♥ ♥

10-12 oz. unsweetened almond, cashew, coconut, or flax milk
2 tbsp. Earthfood Powder
1 tbsp. fresh ground almond or peanut butter
½ tsp. pure vanilla extract
1 tbsp. fresh ginger
1 tsp. cinnamon
Dash of ground nutmeg
½ cup canned chickpeas, rinsed and drained
½ cup frozen organic peaches
¼ of a small avocado, peeled and seeded

Instructions:

Add all ingredients to a high-powered blender (such as Vitamix, Blendtec, or Ninja) in the order listed and blend until smooth.

Nutrition Facts: Calories: 485; Total Fat: 26 g; Saturated Fat: 4 g; Sodium: 790 mg; Potassium: 810 mg; Total Carbohydrates: 47 g; Dietary Fiber: 16 g; Net Carbohydrates: 31 g; Sugar: 5 g (no added sugar); Protein: 20 g

Note: Peace of Health shakes are not sweet, and that is by design. Sweetness is a trained preference, one that can be changed. The goal is to recalibrate your taste buds so that you begin to pick up the natural sweetness of the small amount of fruit in the shakes, without having to add sweetener or extra fruit. For a sweeter shake, refer to the tips offered in the "Do-It-Yourself Shakes" section at the beginning of the book.

Missing Peace #11: Connect to Your Inner Voice

> Silence is a fence around wisdom.
> —German proverb

We all have an inner voice. Some call it intuition, while others refer to it as a gut feeling. Where does this voice come from? I believe it is the voice of my higher self, my true nature. It is a direct link to where I came from before I inhabited this female body of five feet, three inches, with brown eyes. This voice is Divine energy, Source, God,

Nature, Spirit, or whatever you choose to call it. The name doesn't matter. In fact, I find that when we try to label it, we inadvertently negate its immense power. We almost belittle it. The name then conjures up images of something outside of us.

As I contemplate the source of this inner voice, there is a deep knowing that I am directly connected to it. How else am I able to explain unbelievably good ideas that seem to come out of thin air? Where did these hunches and gut feelings come from that sure enough came true? Where does my pure clarity of purpose originate? I have no doubt that what I am doing with my life is exactly what I'm supposed to be doing. I am living my purpose, and I feel it deep within.

As human beings, we have gotten pretty good at ignoring this voice, yet it is essential that you learn how to tap into it. Tune in. When it tells you to go left instead of right, go left; there's a reason. When you have a sure knowing about something but don't know how you know it, that's the voice, so don't question it.

We have a pet box turtle named Dan. This summer, we put him outside in an enclosure that Wayne built for him. He loves the outdoors, so weather permitting, we naturally try to give him as much time outside as possible. One evening, it started to thunderstorm, but we thought nothing of it, because Dan loves being out in the rain. After about thirty minutes, the storm passed, and the sun came out again. It was getting late, and Wayne went to retrieve Dan to put him back in his indoor enclosure. To our surprise, Dan was gone! He escaped and was nowhere to be found. We frantically scoured every square inch of our backyard, searching under countless bushes and leaf piles. No Dan. Wayne was visibly upset and reluctantly suggested we cease our search.

"Mel, let's just let him go," he said. "There's no way we are going to find him out here."

Wayne resignedly threw in the towel, but I continued to search. What he didn't realize was that I had an inner knowing that Dan was close by. I could feel it in my gut. As I tapped into my inner voice, it guided me to go to the edge of our property line. *Go to the back! Go to the back!* I heard it say. I followed these intuitive instructions and continued walking until I reached our neighbor's backyard, some five hundred feet from Dan's enclosure. Sure enough, there he was, frightened and closed up in his shell by the neighbor's fence, almost completely camouflaged by his surroundings. I picked him up, gave him a big hug (yes, it is possible to hug a turtle), and proceeded to share my find with a very jubilant Wayne.

Call it your inner voice or a quiet knowing; we all have it. We just have to get quiet, tune in, and trust.

Meditation: A Tool for Connecting to Your Inner Voice

Why are we so good at ignoring this voice? Quite honestly, I don't believe we even recognize it when it speaks. We may not even know what it is or trust it, for that matter. Or perhaps we're so busy listening to the constant chatter of our egocentric mind that we don't make the peaceful space necessary to hear it.

Meditation is the most effective way I know to tap into my inner voice. In the previous Missing Peace, Live with the End in Mind, you were introduced to a form of visualization called End in Mind (EIM) meditation. The difference between these two meditations is that the goal of the EIM meditation is to visualize yourself as the end product of your desires already manifested, whereas the other is to still your mind. It is during this second meditation where I focus intently on my breath and come into the present moment so that I am able to tap into my inner wisdom.

All of our power resides in the present moment. And because we can't breathe in the past or future, our breath is the perfect opportunity to settle into our body, bring us into the now, and access our Light of Peace.

There is no right way to meditate. For me, I find complete peace during meditation as I envision my Light of Peace, radiating throughout my entire body. This light is my true nature, my connection to Divine energy, and there is a direct link between it and me. In fact, I believe, with every fiber of my being, that I *am* it.

Don't get me wrong; this meditation experience that I am speaking of does not involve stopping thought. That would be impossible, as we have anywhere between fifty thousand and seventy thousand thoughts each day. When a thought creeps into my mind while I'm meditating, I acknowledge it and gently escort it out of my inner space, while continuing to focus on my breath.

During these quiet, meditative moments, I am able to clear the static and make room for my intuitive abilities to surface. I meditate in the morning, about fifteen minutes after waking up. Why? Because I haven't talked to a single person, checked a single email, or allowed any momentum to build. I literally wake up, brush my teeth, take my vitamins, stretch, and meditate.

I invite you to try it out for yourself; experience the peace and power that come from going within. Start with five minutes, and increase your time from there if you choose. You may find it helpful to listen to guided meditations, which walk you through the process step by step. There are a number of free guided meditations available online, or you can download one of the many meditation apps available through your phone.

Meditation and Healthy Choices

You may be wondering what meditation has to do with making positive lifestyle choices. First, meditation is, in and of itself, a healthy choice. It lowers blood pressure, reduces stress, and provides you with a calm and easy state of mind. But I would like to take this even deeper, if I may.

Your higher self knows what is best for your health. It is grounded in purity and nature, and it knows how to thrive.

And since it comes from nature, does it not make logical sense that it would desire sustenance from the same source?

Deep inside of us is a constant craving to feel good and at peace, but we often lose touch and forget what good and peace feel like. You know exactly what I'm talking about if, right now, you are reading these words, knowing that things must change for you. You know that you deserve more and better than what you've been feeding yourself.

I fully respect the fact that it's not so easy to just say no to your kryptonite food, to rationalize and think it through when you're faced with it. Food is legal, it's delicious, and (depending on what and how much you eat) it can contribute to ease or dis-ease in your body. The point is, food will always be around; there's no escaping it, so you must learn how to coexist with it peacefully if you want to heal and live from your higher self.

Not too long ago, I was trying to explain to a client how to walk away from tempting foods. I said, "Look at the food; tell yourself you can have it if you really want it, and then return to your why statement, which is, why am I choosing to make healthier choices for myself?" I would continue by saying, "Once you train your body to eat healthy food, it will crave it."

This wisdom is still true today, but there was something missing in my advice. I discovered that once my clients made the declaration that no food was forbidden, thus removing the power from their kryptonite food, they would initially be at ease, and for the first time in their lives, the heavy weight of food was lifted off their shoulders. They were at peace. But to my frustration, I would soon learn that they were still eating those foods, the very same foods that caused problems to begin with. What was I missing here? How is it that I was able to master such control over food all of these years, and yet my advice to these clients I loved so much felt incomplete? It was as if I got them excited with a glimpse of peace, only to disappoint them when they weren't able to sustain the control.

The missing link to this permanent peace can be described as follows: I had—and still have, to this day—an unspoken power that, at the time, couldn't be put into words. I was tapping into and listening to what my higher self desired, only I wasn't conscious of it. This power enabled me to walk past a box of fresh doughnuts, the food that used to leave me powerless and weak in the knees, and not feel tempted to take one. This invisible force empowered me to say no to the pizza in favor of a veggie tray at a holiday party. Sure, I eat a doughnut once a year on my birthday, and I enjoy a square or two of chocolate several times a week; the difference is, now I am fully conscious of the choice I am making. This consciousness is represented by my inner voice, the observer that only knows wellness. And when I tap into it, making the healthy choice is incredibly effortless.

I believe that when my battle with binge eating disorder came to a breaking point, a crack was created that allowed my higher self to shine through, revealing a ray of light where there was once only darkness. It's as if Divine energy decided that I received everything I needed out of the eating disorder, and it was time for healing, for the next phase of my journey. I've come to the enlightened realization that my Light of Peace was there all along, I was just looking in all the wrong places.

You too can tap into your inner voice and access the power to heal your negative relationship with food and build healthy habits for life. It is during daily meditation and quiet reflection, where you are able to reach that place inside you that will settle for nothing less than purity. When you connect to this deeper you, really settle in and listen, choosing veggies over pizza will feel like home.

Make Peace Exercise: Connect to Your Inner Voice

After completing your morning End in Mind meditation, take another five minutes to practice living in the present moment by settling into your body and following your breath. Pay attention to signs that your inner voice is trying to speak to you. They can come in the form of good ideas, hunches, gut feelings, or simply a quiet knowing.

Return to Your Light of Peace

You have the ability to access your inner voice any time you choose. Tapping into this inner wisdom is especially powerful when making choices for your well-being. Simply get quiet and breathe into your Light of Peace. Then listen, trust, and decide.

Recommended Peace of Health Shake

Chocolate Mint Shake

6 Earthfood Servings ♥♥♥♥♥♥

12 oz. unsweetened almond, cashew, coconut, or flax milk
2 tbsp. Earthfood Powder
½ of a small avocado, peeled and seeded
½ banana, frozen
1 tbsp. raw cacao powder
½ tsp. pure peppermint extract or paste
2 cups fresh organic spinach

Instructions:

Add all ingredients to a high-powered blender (such as Vitamix, Blendtec, or Ninja) in the order listed and blend until smooth.

Nutrition Facts: Calories: 380; Total Fat: 25 g; Saturated Fat: 10 g; Sodium: 210 mg; Potassium: 990 mg; Total Carbohydrates: 32 g; Dietary Fiber: 14 g; Net Carbohydrates: 18 g; Sugar: 8 g (no added sugar); Protein: 13 g

Note: Peace of Health shakes are not sweet, and that is by design. Sweetness is a trained preference, one that can be changed. The goal is to recalibrate your taste buds so that you begin to pick up the natural sweetness of the small amount of fruit in the shakes, without having to add sweetener or extra fruit. For a sweeter shake, refer to the tips offered in the "Do-It-Yourself Shakes" section at the beginning of the book.

Closing

Rest in Living Peace

> Don't fight darkness; bring the light,
> and darkness will disappear.
> —Maharishi Mahesh Yogi

As I reflect back over my life up until this very moment, I have zero regrets. I believe with every fiber of my being that every challenge that confronted me was by perfect design. The binge eating disorder provided me with experiences that I never would've consciously signed up for, and because I did everything wrong, I learned the lessons necessary to write this book. Of course, I didn't see it at the time because I was too busy fighting for my life.

These eleven Missing Peaces provide me with a great deal of comfort as I move through this wild ride called life. I feel empowered beyond explanation, to realize that I am the creator of my life, the artist of my story, with a brush in one hand and a palette of vibrant colors in the other. Before me lies a blank canvas on which I am free to paint any picture

I desire. I choose a woman whose health is supreme, with a body full of energy and a life full of purpose, confidence, bliss, and peace. But wait. As I take a step back and look at my freshly painted canvas, I realize this landscape looks an awful lot like me already. Could it be that my vision is not a vision after all, but rather me in living, breathing form? The real deal? Am I actually *her* already? Yes, when I allow it. And when I allow it, I feel on purpose.

Oh, what a wonderful life this is, to know that the only thing required of me to step into the person I already am and live the life of my dreams is to be fully present for this moment and breathe into my Light of Peace, my higher self. I think I can handle that.

Now, what about you, dear friend? You are no different. I need you to understand that you don't have to physically die to rest in the peace that is your birthright. No matter what your current situation, you hold within you the power to peace. If you can imagine your healthiest self and feel it within, it will manifest because it is the law.

Surely, some days you may not believe this, especially if your present-day life lacks any evidence of health. The truth is, we are all made up of cracks, some the size of the Grand Canyon, others nearly microscopic. These cracks can take on the form of disease, food addiction, or undesirable lab values, and at first glance, they appear to us as misfortune. But don't be fooled. Our cracks are genuine gifts. We're so quick to fill them in with hopeless thoughts, a sugary treat, greasy comfort food, a glass of wine, or bitter, self-blaming words; after all, they are cracks and in need of repair (as if any one of these adhesives can actually fix the crack).

Consider this: What if the way to inner peace and a life full of good health is *through* your cracks? When you surrender and embrace them, you allow your Light of Peace to penetrate through, shining a bright beam on who you really are and what you are capable of. From this place, you are in a receiving mode, and all of a sudden, solutions come to you that in the past couldn't get through. Why? Because they can only reach you through your cracks.

I think Josh Groban captures beautifully what I am trying to say here, with the following verse from his song "Let Me Fall":

> The one I want
> The one I will become
> Will catch me

To experience the song in all of its glory, I strongly encourage you to do an internet search for the video. Be prepared with tissues in hand.

All you have to do is *want* to feel better more than you've wanted anything. Self-love is important here. I realize that may be a far reach for many, especially if the thought of even looking at yourself in the mirror is enough to send you running for the hills.

Let's start with acquaintances. Surely you lend a bit of friendliness to your current acquaintances, be they work or social. You hold no harm for them. You can smile at them with ease; in fact, you may find that you really like them and wouldn't mind getting to know them better.

Next, move to friends. Take yourself out for a cup of coffee and notice how lovely it is to be with you. Now, let's gently move to love. Feel your way into it, and allow yourself to fall madly in love with the real you. I think you will be surprised to find that you didn't even have to try because the love was there all along.

Be still and listen for your inner voice. Let go and allow it to guide you. You will know you're on the right track because it will feel right. Be sure to breathe into your Light of Peace and check in every step along your journey, exploring your thoughts and feelings. Do they match up to what you are getting out of life? Are you getting closer to or further away from your highest, healthiest vision of yourself?

Trust your emotions and choose peace whenever you can: a peaceful thought, word, feeling, food choice. How does that choice feel? Peaceful or restrictive? On purpose or off? When you feel off course, this is your cue to make a gentle shift in your thoughts, feelings, and actions toward peace. How do you feel now?

My one true wish for you is this, dear friend: When you meet with your final hours on this earthly plane, you will have no regrets. Not one. My hope is that you allowed yourself to embody your highest vision of you and lived a life true to yourself. Most of all, I wish that you let yourself be happy and at peace, because both are a choice.

Remember Bronnie Ware, author of *The Top Five Regrets of the Dying*? As revealed in her book, the fifth regret was: I wish that I had let myself be happier.

What are you waiting for? Go ahead. Give yourself permission to live the picture of health you so masterfully created. This is your picture, your life, your masterpiece. Remember, you already *are* the product of your wildest dreams. You already *are* the end. Let your light shine bright and step into the real you, the one that has been patiently and lovingly waiting for your arrival.

Recipes

Peace of Health Shakes

All of my Peace of Health shakes call for Earthfood Powder, a homemade plant-based protein powder that is both economical and easy to prepare. The recipe is listed below.

Note: Peace of Health shakes are not sweet, and that is by design. Sweetness is a trained preference, one that can be changed. The goal is to recalibrate your taste buds so that you begin to pick up the natural sweetness of the small amount of fruit in the shakes, without having to add sweetener or extra fruit.

For a sweeter shake, try adding one of the following:

- a natural flavor enhancer like a few dashes of ground cinnamon; a wedge of lemon, lime, or orange; a few sprigs of fresh mint; or a teaspoon of organic, pure vanilla or peppermint extract

- ¼–½ cup more fruit
- up to 1 tsp. of raw honey, pure maple syrup, or coconut nectar, or one pitted date

Instructions for Preparing All Peace of Health Shakes

Add all ingredients to a high-powered blender (such as Vitamix, Blendtec, or Ninja) in the order listed and blend until smooth.

Earthfood Powder

2 Earthfoods per servings ♥ ♥

Serving size: 2 tbsp.
1 cup raw pepitas
1 cup hemp hearts
1 cup milled flaxseed
1 tbsp. ground cinnamon
1 tbsp. raw cacao powder
1 tsp. sea salt
1 cup Bob's Red Mill Pea Protein Powder

Instructions:

Add pepitas through sea salt to a food processor (or blender) and process until seeds are broken down (about 1 minute). Pour contents into a large mixing bowl or container with lid and add pea protein, mixing/shaking until thoroughly combined. Store in airtight container in refrigerator or freezer.

Nutrition Facts per serving (2 tbsp.): Calories: 100; Total Fat: 7 g; Saturated Fat: 1 g; Sodium: 150 mg; Potassium: 0 mg; Total Carbohydrates: 3 g; Dietary Fiber: 3 g; Net Carbohydrates: 0 g; Sugar: 0 g; Protein: 8 g

Chocolate Almond Cherry Shake

6 Earthfood Servings ♥♥♥♥♥♥

10–12 oz. unsweetened almond, cashew, coconut, or flax milk
2 tbsp. Earthfood Powder
1 tbsp. raw cacao powder
1 tbsp. fresh ground almond butter
1 cup frozen organic cherries

Nutrition Facts: Calories: 385; Total Fat: 23 g; Saturated Fat: 8 g; Sodium: 160 mg; Potassium: 180 mg; Total Carbohydrates: 36 g; Dietary Fiber: 11 g; Net Carbohydrates: 25 g; Sugar: 19 g (no added sugar); Protein: 14 g

Clean and Green Shake

6 Earthfood Servings ♥ ♥ ♥ ♥ ♥ ♥

10 oz. unsweetened almond, cashew, coconut, or flax milk
2 tbsp. Earthfood Powder

½–1 tsp. matcha
½ tbsp. MCT oil
½ of a small avocado, peeled and seeded
2 cups fresh organic spinach
½ cup frozen mango
¼ lemon with rind

Nutrition Facts: Calories: 400; Total Fat: 31 g; Saturated Fat: 15 g; Sodium: 200 mg; Potassium: 930 mg; Total Carbohydrates: 31 g; Dietary Fiber: 15 g; Net Carbohydrates: 16 g; Sugar: 12 g (no added sugar); Protein: 14 g

Ginger Pear Shake

7 Earthfood Servings ♥♥♥♥♥♥♥

10 oz. unsweetened almond, cashew, coconut, or flax milk
2 tbsp. Earthfood Powder
1 tbsp. fresh ginger
½ tsp. cinnamon
1 tbsp. coconut butter
½ cup carrots
1 cup fresh sliced organic pears (with skin on; about one small pear)

Nutrition Facts: Calories: 375; Total Fat: 23 g; Saturated Fat: 15 g; Sodium: 200 mg; Potassium: 490 mg; Total Carbohydrates: 38 g; Dietary Fiber: 14 g; Net Carbohydrates: 24 g; Sugar: 20 g (no added sugar); Protein: 10 g

Tropical Turmeric Shake

7 Earthfood Servings ❤❤❤❤❤❤❤

12 oz. unsweetened coconut milk
2 tbsp. Earthfood Powder
¼ lime, with rind
1 tbsp. fresh turmeric
1 tbsp. fresh ginger
¼ of a small avocado, peeled and seeded
½ tbsp. MCT oil
2 cups fresh organic spinach or kale
¼ cup frozen pineapple
¼ frozen banana or ¼ cup frozen mango

Organic, unsweetened coconut flakes (sprinkled on top of prepared smoothie)

Nutrition Facts: Calories: 400; Total Fat: 30 g; Saturated Fat: 15 g; Sodium: 190 mg; Potassium: 540 mg; Total Carbohydrates: 34 g; Dietary Fiber: 11 g; Net Carbohydrates: 23 g; Sugar: 10 g (no added sugar); Protein: 13 g

Healthy Brain Shake

7 Earthfood Servings ❤❤❤❤❤❤❤

12 oz. unsweetened almond, cashew, coconut, or flax milk
2 tbsp. Earthfood Powder
½ tbsp. MCT oil
⅛ cup walnuts

¼ of a small avocado, peeled and seeded
1 tbsp. fresh turmeric
2 cups fresh organic spinach or kale
½ cup frozen wild blueberries
¼ lemon with rind

Nutrition Facts: Calories: 460; Total Fat: 36 g; Saturated Fat: 9 g; Sodium: 490 mg; Potassium: 750 mg; Total Carbohydrates: 30 g; Dietary Fiber: 12 g; Net Carbohydrates: 18 g; Sugar: 7 g (no added sugar); Protein: 16 g

Gut-Loving Chocolate Peanut Butter Shake

5 Earthfood Servings ♥ ♥ ♥ ♥ ♥

2 oz. plain, whole milk kefir (if dairy-intolerant, omit and use a total of 12 oz. of unsweetened nut milk instead)
8 oz. unsweetened almond, cashew, coconut, or flax milk
2 tbsp. Earthfood Powder
1 tbsp. raw cacao powder
1 tbsp. fresh ground peanut butter
1 tsp. pure vanilla extract
½ banana, ripe (frozen makes it creamier!)
¼ of a small avocado, peeled and seeded

Nutrition Facts: Calories: 435; Total Fat: 29 g; Saturated Fat: 10 g; Sodium: 250 mg; Potassium: 450 mg; Total Carbohydrates: 32 g; Dietary Fiber: 11 g; Net Carbohydrates: 21 g; Sugar: 10 g (no added sugar); Protein: 17 g

Berry Power Shake

6 Earthfood Servings ❤❤❤❤❤❤

12 oz. unsweetened almond, cashew, coconut, or flax milk
2 tbsp. Earthfood Powder
1 tbsp. chia seeds
¼ small avocado, peeled and seeded
½ tbsp. coconut butter
½ tbsp. fresh ground almond butter
¼ lemon with rind
½ cup frozen wild blueberries
½ cup frozen cranberries

Nutrition Facts: Calories: 440; Total Fat: 31 g; Saturated Fat: 7 g; Sodium: 460 mg; Potassium: 700 mg; Total Carbohydrates: 35 g; Dietary Fiber: 20 g; Net Carbohydrates: 15 g; Sugar: 9 g (no added sugar); Protein: 16 g

Strawberry Lemon Surprise Shake

7 Earthfood Servings ❤❤❤❤❤❤❤

12–16 oz. unsweetened almond, cashew, coconut, or flax milk
2 tbsp. Earthfood Powder
¼ of a small avocado, peeled and seeded
1 cup fresh organic kale
1 cup shredded red cabbage
1 tbsp. fresh ginger
¼ of a lemon, with rind

½ cup frozen cauliflower (surprise)
½ cup frozen organic strawberries

Nutrition Facts: Calories: 320; Total Fat: 20 g; Saturated Fat: 8 g; Sodium: 200 mg; Potassium: 680 mg; Total Carbohydrates: 31 g; Dietary Fiber: 14 g; Net Carbohydrates: 17 g; Sugar: 8 g (no added sugar); Protein: 13 g

Melanie's Go-To Power Shake

8 Earthfood Servings ♥♥♥♥♥♥♥♥

12 oz. unsweetened almond, cashew, coconut, or flax milk
1 tsp. maca powder
2 tbsp. Earthfood Powder
¼ lemon with rind
1 tbsp. fresh ginger
1 tbsp. fresh turmeric
½ of a small avocado, peeled and seeded
2 cups fresh organic kale
½ cup frozen wild blueberries

Nutrition Facts: Calories: 400; Total Fat: 29 g; Saturated Fat: 9 g; Sodium: 195 mg; Potassium: 685 mg; Total Carbohydrates: 40 g; Dietary Fiber: 16 g; Net Carbohydrates: 24 g; Sugar: 8 g (no added sugar); Protein: 14 g

Peachy Keen Shake

7 Earthfood Servings ♥♥♥♥♥♥♥

10–12 oz. unsweetened almond, cashew, coconut, or flax milk

2 tbsp. Earthfood Powder

1 tbsp. fresh ground almond or peanut butter

½ tsp. pure vanilla extract

1 tbsp. fresh ginger

1 tsp. cinnamon

Dash of ground nutmeg

½ cup canned chickpeas, rinsed and drained

½ cup frozen organic peaches

¼ of a small avocado, peeled and seeded

Nutrition Facts: Calories: 485; Total Fat: 26 g; Saturated Fat: 4 g; Sodium: 790 mg; Potassium: 810 mg; Total Carbohydrates: 47 g; Dietary Fiber: 16 g; Net Carbohydrates: 31 g; Sugar: 5 g (no added sugar); Protein: 20 g

Chocolate Mint Shake

6 Earthfood Servings ♥ ♥ ♥ ♥ ♥ ♥

12 oz. unsweetened almond, cashew, coconut, or flax milk

2 tbsp. Earthfood Powder

½ of a small avocado, peeled and seeded

½ banana, frozen

1 tbsp. raw cacao powder

½ tsp. pure peppermint extract or paste

2 cups fresh organic spinach

Nutrition Facts: Calories: 380; Total Fat: 25 g; Saturated Fat: 10 g; Sodium: 210 mg; Potassium: 990 mg; Total Carbohydrates: 32 g; Dietary Fiber: 14 g; Net Carbohydrates: 18 g; Sugar: 8 g (no added sugar); Protein: 13 g

Appendix

Earthfoods

Planning healthy meals is key to creating healthy food cravings. I only have one rule when it comes to meal planning: Build your meals to include a minimum of three servings of Earthfoods. Three is the magic number to turn any meal into a PeaceMeal.

Earthfoods are single-ingredient plant foods that are powerful beyond measure; they can heal your body at a cellular level. They are the foods your body was designed to eat and truly longs for.

Vegetables
One serving of Earthfood = 1 cup raw or cooked; 2 cups leafy greens

Artichoke
Arugula
Asparagus
Beets

Bok choy
Broccoli
Broccoli rabe
Brussels sprouts
Cabbage
Carrots
Cauliflower
Celery (organic)
Chard
Chive
Collard greens
Cucumbers
Dandelion greens
Eggplant
Endive
Fennel
Garlic
Green beans
Jicama
Kale
Kohlrabi
Leeks
Mushrooms
Mustard greens
Okra
Onion
Parsnips
Peppers (organic)
Potato (organic)
Radicchio
Radish

Rhubarb
Rutabaga
Scallions
Shallots
Snap peas
Snow peas
Spinach (organic)
Squash: acorn, butternut, spaghetti, pumpkin
Sweet potato/yam
Tomatillo
Tomato (organic)
Turnip greens
Turnips
Watercress
Zucchini

Fruit
One serving of Earthfood = ½ cup (no juice)

Apple (organic)
Apricots
Banana
Blackberries
Blueberries
Boysenberries
Cherries (organic)
Cranberries
Dragon fruit
Elderberries
Figs
Goji berries

Grapefruit

Grapes (organic)

Guava

Jackfruit

Kiwi

Lemon

Lime

Mango

Melon: cantaloupe, honeydew, watermelon

Mulberries

Nectarine (organic)

Orange: blood orange, clementine, Mandarin, tangerine

Papaya

Passion fruit

Peach (organic)

Pear (organic)

Persimmon

Pineapple

Plantain

Plum

Pomegranate seeds

Quince

Raspberries

Star fruit

Strawberries (organic)

Ugli fruit

Legumes
One serving of Earthfood = ½ cup cooked

Adzuki beans
Black beans
Black-eyed peas
Edamame (organic)
Garbanzo beans
Kidney beans
Lentils: green, red
Lima beans
Mung beans
Navy beans
Pinto beans
Peanuts: ¼ cup
Peas
Red beans

Healthy Fats
One serving of Earthfood = ¼ cup of these nuts/seeds

Almonds
Brazil nuts
Cashews
Hazelnuts (filberts)
Macadamia nuts
Pecans
Pine nuts
Pistachios
Pumpkin seeds
Sacha inchi seeds
Sunflower seeds

Walnuts

One serving of Earthfood = 1 tbsp. of these seeds

Chia seeds
Flaxseed (ground)
Hemp seeds
Sesame seeds

Other
One serving of Earthfood equals

Avocado: ½ of a small; ¼ of large
Nut/seed butter (peanut, almond, cashew, macadamia nut, sunflower, etc.): 1 tbsp.
Coconut: 2-inch piece fresh coconut; 2 tbsp. unsweetened, shredded coconut; 1 tbsp. virgin, unrefined coconut oil; 1 tbsp. coconut butter

Functional Foods

One serving of Earthfood = 1 tsp. dried or 1 tbsp. fresh herbs/spices

Basil
Cilantro
Dill
Garlic
Ginger
Lavender
Mint

Oregano
Parsley
Rosemary
Saffron
Sage
Thyme
Turmeric

Other
One serving of Earthfood equals

Green tea: 1 bag or 1 tbsp. loose tea
Matcha tea: ½ tsp.
Cacao: 1 tbsp.
Maca: 1 tsp.
Wheatgrass: ¼ tsp powder; 1 oz. juice

Product Recommendation List

Cacao Powder: Navitas
Chia Seeds: Bob's Red Mill; Navitas
Coconut Butter: Artisana
Coconut Cream: Let's Do Organic Creamed Coconut
Coconut Flakes/Shredded: Let's Do Organic
Coconut Milk, canned: Native Forest Simple Organic Unsweetened Coconut Milk
Coconut Nectar: Big Tree Farms, Coconut Secret
Coconut Oil, organic and unrefined: Spectrum, Carrington Farms, Nutiva
Flaxseed: Bob's Red Mill
Ginger powder: Organic Traditions

Greens powder: Axe Organics Organic SuperGreens

Hemp hearts: Navitas

Honey, organic and raw: Madhava; Wholesome

Kefir: Wallaby Organic Plain Whole Milk Kefir

Maca powder: Navitas

Maple syrup, pure: choose Grade A Dark Color and Robust Flavor

Matcha: Nutritional Roots; Navitas

MCT oil: Bulletproof Brain Octane Oil

Nut/seed butters (almond, cashew, peanut, macadamia, sunflower, pistachio, etc.): Look for brands offering maximum of two ingredients: nuts/seeds and salt

Nut milks, unsweetened: Elmhurst Unsweetened Milked Almonds

Peppermint extract: Flavorganics

Protein powders:

> Ancient Nutrition Bone Broth Protein (Pure, Greens or Turmeric); Garden of Life Raw Organic Protein (Unflavored); Sprout Living Epic Protein (Original); Sprout Living Sunflower Seed Protein; Sprout Living Pumpkin Seed Protein; Bob's Red Mill Pea Protein Powder

Turmeric powder: Navitas; Organic Traditions

Vanilla extract: Flavorganics

Wheatgrass: Navitas

Bibliography

Preface

Ware, Bronnie. "Regrets of the Dying." Bronnie Ware, www.bronnieware.com/blog/regrets-of-the-dying.

Missing Peace #4:

Dyer, Wayne W. *Excuses Begone!: How to Change Lifelong, Self-Defeating Thinking Habits.* Hay House, 2012, p. 35.

Missing Peace #5:

Fondin, Michelle. "Portion Control: How Much Are You Actually Eating?" The Chopra Center. www.chopra.com/articles/portion-control-how-much-are-you-actually-eating#sm.00000r8vkaixwtf2espkf75ybj0a2.

Missing Peace #6:

"What Is Celiac Disease?" Celiac Disease Foundation, celiac.org/celiac-disease/understanding-celiac-disease-2/what-is-celiac-disease/

Avena, Nicole M., et al. "Evidence for Sugar Addiction: Behavioral and Neurochemical Effects of Intermittent, Excessive Sugar Intake." Neuroscience and Biobehavioral Reviews, US National Library of Medicine, 2008, www.ncbi.nlm.nih.gov/pmc/articles/PMC2235907/.

Breus, Michael J. "The Connection Between Sleep and Appetite." *Psychology Today*, October 29, 2013, www.psychologytoday.com/blog/sleep-newzzz/201310/the-connection-between-sleep-and-appetite.

Gunnars, Kris. "Leptin and Leptin Resistance: Everything You Need to Know." Healthline, Healthline Media, June 4, 2017, www.healthline.com/nutrition/leptin-101#section5.

Kilroy, Dana Sullivan. "Cravings Could Be Defeated with Two Little Words." *Los Angeles Times*, July 21, 2012, articles.latimes.com/2012/jul/21/health/la-he-cravings-20120721.

Mercola, Joseph. "What Happens in Your Body When You Eat Too Much Sugar?" Mercola.com, articles.mercola.com/sugar-side-effects.aspx.

Mowll, Brian. "Artificial Sweeteners Are Not So Sweet." January 26, 2018, drmowll.com/artificial-sweeteners-are-not-so-sweet/.

Sisson, Mark. "16 Things That Affect Your Gut Bacteria." Mark's Daily Apple, September 16, 2016, www.marksdailyapple.com/16-things-that-affect-your-gut-bacteria/.

Williams, David. "Gut Bacteria May Influence Food Cravings." www.drdavidwilliams.com/gut-bacteria-may-influence-food-cravings/.

Williams, David. "The Role of Prebiotics in Maintaining Healthy Gut Flora." www.drdavidwilliams.com/the-role-of-prebiotics-in-maintaining-healthy-gut-flora/.

Williams, David. "Lifestyle Habits That Damage Gut Bacteria." www.drdavidwilliams.com/lifestyle-habits-that-damage-gut-bacteria/.

Yang, Qing. "Gain Weight by 'Going Diet'? Artificial Sweeteners and the Neurobiology of Sugar Cravings." *The Yale Journal of Biology and Medicine,* June 2010, www.ncbi.nlm.nih.gov/pmc/articles/PMC2892765/.

Missing Peace #8:

Emoto, Masaru. "What Is the Photograph of Frozen Water Crystals?" www.masaru-emoto.net/english/water-crystal.html.

"*The Guest House* by Mewlana Jalaluddin Rumi." *Famous Poems, Famous Poets.* allpoetry.com/poem/8534703-The-Guest-House-by-Mewlana-Jalaluddin-Rumi.

Lipton, Bruce. "What Is Epigenetics?" July 15, 2014, www.brucelipton.com/blog/what-epigenetics.

Lipton, Bruce. "What Thoughts and Emotions Are Affecting Your Cells? Here Is the Science Behind It." August 28, 2014, www.brucelipton.com/blog/what-thoughts-and-emotions-are-affecting-your-cells-here-the-science-behind-it.

Hicks, Esther, and Jerry Hicks. *Ask and It Is Given: Learning to Manifest Your Desires*. Hay House Publications, 2004.

Stanford University. "Text of Steve Jobs' Commencement Address (2005)." Stanford News, 12 June 2017, news.stanford.edu/2005/06/14/jobs-061505/.

Missing Peace #10:

Peer, Marisa. "Train Your Brain To Do What You Want." Mindvalley Academy, www.mindvalleyacademy.com/blog/mind/train-your-brain.

Index

A

Abraham Hicks 106, 117, 119
A Course in Miracles 2
acute inflammation 44, 45
addiction 16, 21, 33, 71, 109,
    136, 156, 180
alcohol xxiv, 69, 81, 82, 87
alignment xii, 4, 27
allowed xl, 23, 24, 25, 27, 148,
    150, 158
    allowing xxxvii, xxxviii,
        xlii, xliii, 1, 3, 5,
        8, 21, 26, 116, 117,
        118, 121
almond xiv, xvi, xvii, 9, 22,
    28, 36, 38, 63, 89, 95,
    96, 100, 101, 122, 128,
    143, 152, 163, 164, 165,
    166, 167, 168, 169, 175,
    176, 178
    almond butter xiv, 9, 95,
        96, 101, 163, 167
anchoring xxxvii, xxxix, xliii,
    13, 103

anger 4
antibiotics 77
antioxidants 43, 47, 68, 69
appetite xxi, xxiv, 61, 78, 80,
    81, 86, 87, 180
    appetite scale 61
apple xvii, 26, 39, 40, 42, 43,
    47, 76, 77, 96, 173, 180
apple cider vinegar 76, 77
artificial food coloring 77
artificial sweeteners xvi, 15, 16,
    42, 68, 69, 77, 79, 80,
    81, 87, 95, 180, 181
arugula 36, 40, 171
ask and allow 117
aspartame xvi, 15, 80
attachment 110, 116, 121
attitude 133, 140
avocados xiv, xvi, xvii, xviii,
    xxx, 19, 22, 33, 34, 36,
    40, 47, 53, 64, 69, 79,
    89, 96, 101, 122, 128,
    141, 143, 152, 164, 165,
    166, 167, 168, 169, 176

avocado xiv, xvi, xvii,
xviii, 19, 22, 33,
36, 40, 53, 64, 89,
96, 101, 122, 128,
141, 143, 152, 164,
165, 166, 167, 168,
169, 176
awaken to the source of your
unsupportive cravings
xlii, 42, 67, 68, 91
awareness xli, 31, 62, 84, 85,
108, 121, 135
Awesomeness Fest 138
Ayurveda 59

B

babies xli, 54, 55, 56, 58, 84
baby xli, 40, 54, 55, 56,
58, 61, 83, 84, 85,
86, 94, 95
bacteria 74, 75, 76, 77, 79,
180, 181
banana xvii, 26, 53, 76, 89,
152, 165, 166, 169, 173
beans xv, 36, 47, 76, 172, 175
beef xxii, 41, 48, 79
beer 42, 82
beliefs x, xxvii, xxviii, xlii,
xliii, 3, 24, 50, 51, 103,
111, 112, 113, 114
believing xii, xxxvii, xlii,
xliv, 103, 131, 138
berries xiv, xvii, 38, 47, 96, 173
berry power shake 100, 167

binge eating disorder xii, xxv,
xxxv, 71, 77, 107, 109,
150, 155
binges xi, xii, xxv, xxviii, xxix,
xxx, xxxi, xxxv, 16, 38,
69, 71, 77, 107, 109,
150, 155
binge xi, xii, xxv, xxviii,
xxix, xxx, xxxi,
xxxv, 16, 38, 69,
71, 77, 107, 109,
150, 155
binging xxx, xxxvi, 15, 17,
71, 109
bliss xii, xiii, 4, 27, 118, 156
blood sugar xvi, xxxii, 2,
15, 19, 28, 41, 44, 46,
47, 48, 56, 69, 72, 81,
82, 136
blueberries xxx, 27, 33, 36, 38,
43, 64, 76, 77, 96, 101,
128, 166, 167, 168, 173
body iii, ix, xiii, xv, xxiii, xxiv,
xxv, xxvi, xxvii, xxviii,
xxix, xxx, xxxi, xxxii,
xxxv, xxxvi, xxxviii,
xxxix, xl, xli, xlii, xliii,
xliv, xlv, 3, 5, 7, 8, 9, 13,
15, 18, 19, 20, 21, 24,
26, 27, 28, 31, 32, 33,
34, 35, 37, 41, 42, 43,
44, 45, 46, 49, 51, 52,
55, 56, 57, 58, 60, 61,
62, 63, 68, 69, 72, 73,
74, 75, 76, 77, 78, 79,
81, 82, 87, 89, 90, 91,

92, 93, 94, 98, 99, 108, 109, 110, 112, 113, 116, 117, 120, 121, 124, 131, 132, 133, 134, 136, 139, 140, 141, 144, 147, 149, 151, 156, 171, 180

body fat 78

brain xxvii, 16, 33, 34, 35, 41, 58, 63, 72, 73, 78, 112, 113, 138, 165, 178, 182

brain fog 35

breakfast xiv, xv, xxiv, xxix, 33, 35, 38, 39, 62, 77, 134, 141

breathe xxxix, 6, 9, 26, 28, 89, 135, 143, 147, 152, 156, 158

breath xxxviii, xliv, 1, 6, 7, 8, 9, 21, 52, 63, 84, 89, 94, 97, 99, 100, 121, 131, 135, 136, 142, 147, 148, 151

broccoli 27, 33, 38, 40, 41, 76, 79, 95, 140, 172

Bronnie Ware xi, 159, 179

Bruce Lipton 111

Brussels sprouts 33, 38, 40, 41, 95, 172

Buddha xxxvi, 104, 106

C

cabbage xviii, 122, 167, 172

cacao xviii, xix, 9, 33, 34, 89, 95, 152, 162, 163, 166, 169, 177

cacao powder xviii, xix, 9, 33, 89, 152, 162, 163, 166, 169, 177

calorie-controlled crap foods 18

CCF 18, 19

calories xix, xxiii, xxvi, xxviii, xxix, xxx, 10, 15, 16, 17, 18, 19, 20, 21, 22, 29, 48, 53, 58, 64, 73, 79, 80, 87, 90, 101, 122, 129, 144, 152, 163, 164, 165, 166, 167, 168, 169, 170

cancer 44, 49

carbohydrate-based 47

career 108, 120, 121

Carl Jung 14

carrots xvii, xviii, 29, 40, 52, 76, 87, 94, 95, 164, 172

cauliflower xvii, xviii, 33, 41, 76, 95, 122, 168, 172

celery 40, 56, 94, 95, 172

celiac disease 70, 179

Celiac Disease Foundation 70, 179

cherries 9, 76, 163, 173

chia seeds xiv, xvi, xvii, 36, 101, 167, 176, 177

chicken 35, 40, 41, 48, 126

chickpeas 95, 96, 143, 169

chocolate xxx, 9, 24, 25, 32, 34, 71, 72, 83, 84, 89, 91, 92, 95, 96, 98, 150, 152, 163, 166, 169

chocolate almond cherry shake
9, 163
chocolate mint shake 152, 169
choose carefully the words
following "I am" xii,
xiii, xxvi, xxxii, xxxvi,
xliii, 3, 6, 23, 35, 37,
38, 57, 86, 91, 94, 103,
113, 119, 123, 124, 125,
126, 127, 133, 139, 141,
142, 145, 147, 148, 150,
155, 157
chronic inflammation 44, 45,
46, 52
cinnamon xviii, xix, 29, 33, 39,
143, 161, 162, 164, 169
clarity 4, 27, 34, 106, 118, 145
classical music 119
clean & green shake 22
clean-plate club xxii
clinging 114, 115, 116, 121
coconut xvi, xvii, xviii, xix, 9,
22, 28, 29, 36, 39, 53,
63, 79, 89, 96, 100, 101,
122, 128, 143, 152, 162,
163, 164, 165, 166, 167,
168, 169, 176, 177
coconut butter 29, 101,
164, 167, 176, 177
coconut milk xvi, xix, 53,
165, 177
complacency x, 20
confidence 4, 37, 156
connect xxxv, xliv, xlv, 18, 28,
85, 107, 131, 144, 151

connecting xxxvii, xxxviii,
xli, xliv, xlv, 1, 106,
131, 146
connect to your inner voice
xliv, 131, 144, 151
conscious breathing 52
conscious breath xxxviii,
1, 6, 7
conscious breaths xxxviii,
1, 6, 7, 28, 128
consistency 9, 35
contemplation x
contrast 4, 107, 108, 109, 111,
112, 117, 118, 119, 132
control xiii, xxxi, xxxiii, xxxv,
xl, xlii, 5, 15, 21, 25,
31, 46, 48, 67, 71, 75,
77, 78, 93, 94, 112,
113, 114, 119, 125, 137,
150, 179
cracks 150, 156, 157
cranberries 76, 101, 167, 173
cravings xvii, xxx, xxxi, xxxii,
xxxvi, xxxvii, xxxix, xli,
xlii, xlv, 15, 19, 32, 33,
37, 38, 42, 44, 67, 68,
69, 73, 74, 75, 77, 78,
79, 80, 86, 87, 89, 91,
92, 93, 94, 95, 97, 99,
100, 149, 171, 180, 181
crave xv, xxix, xxx, xxxii,
xl, 27, 31, 32, 33,
34, 35, 37, 41, 42,
43, 46, 49, 51, 52,
72, 75, 79, 80, 81,

90, 91, 92, 134,
142, 149
craving xvii, xxx, xxxi,
xxxii, xxxvi, xxxvii,
xxxix, xli, xlii, xlv,
15, 19, 32, 33, 37,
38, 42, 44, 67, 68,
69, 73, 74, 75, 77,
78, 79, 80, 86, 87,
89, 91, 92, 93, 94,
95, 97, 99, 100, 149,
171, 180, 181
creamy 93, 96, 99, 100

D

daily rituals x, xxii
David Katz 73, 91
Deepak Chopra 106
dehydration 60, 68, 69, 73,
81, 87
describe your craving 92,
93, 99
detoxifying 82
diabetes 44, 46, 48, 49, 111
dietetics xxv
digestion xvi, 19, 57, 74
digestive issues 35
disease xii, 44, 45, 46, 49, 70,
74, 107, 136, 156, 179
disharmony xxxviii, 1, 8
Divine energy x, xxxvi, xxxviii,
1, 3, 109, 110, 124, 144,
147, 150
divinity 3
dogma 138

do-it-yourself shakes xvi, 10,
23, 29, 54, 64, 90, 101,
123, 129, 144, 153
dopamine 68, 73
doubt 4, 7, 44, 104, 107, 145

E

Earthfoods xiv, xv, xvi, xvii,
xix, xl, 9, 22, 28, 31, 34,
35, 36, 37, 38, 39, 45,
46, 47, 48, 49, 51, 52,
53, 60, 63, 69, 71, 75,
79, 89, 100, 110, 122,
128, 143, 152, 161, 162,
163, 164, 165, 166, 167,
168, 169, 171, 173, 175,
176, 177
Earthfood powder xvi,
xvii, xix, 9, 22,
28, 36, 53, 63, 89,
100, 122, 128, 143,
152, 161, 162, 163,
164, 165, 166, 167,
168, 169
eating disorder xi, xii, xxv,
xxvii, xxxii, xxxv, xxxvi,
71, 77, 107, 109, 150,
151, 155
eggs xxx, xxxi, 39, 40, 41, 79,
95, 123
emotions xxxviii, xliii, xlv,
1, 4, 7, 83, 84, 85, 86,
108, 109, 112, 115, 116,
118, 121, 125, 127, 158,
181, 182

emotion xxxviii, xliii,
      xlv, 1, 4, 7, 83, 84,
      85, 86, 108, 109,
      112, 115, 116, 118,
      121, 125, 127, 158,
      181, 182
emotional states 4, 5, 7, 9,
      68, 122
end in mind xliv, 131, 132,
      133, 134, 135, 138, 140,
      142, 147, 151
   EIM xliv, 141, 142, 147
   End in Mind (EIM)
      meditation
      xliv, 147
Epictetus 132
epigenetics 111, 112, 181
evaluate your craving 97, 100
excitement 4, 139, 140
Excuses Begone 50, 179
exercise xiv, xxx, xxxix, xl,
      xliii, xlv, 2, 8, 13, 21, 27,
      31, 42, 45, 50, 51, 61,
      62, 85, 86, 87, 97, 99,
      115, 116, 120, 126, 127,
      132, 133, 142, 151

F

false beliefs 3
family relationships 120, 121
fat xvi, xvii, xix, xxv, xxviii,
      xxix, xxx, 10, 15, 19,
      22, 26, 29, 41, 48, 50,
      53, 58, 60, 64, 68, 69,
      72, 73, 78, 79, 80, 90,
      91, 93, 101, 122, 123,
      124, 125, 126, 129, 132,
      133, 144, 152, 163, 164,
      165, 166, 167, 168, 169,
      170, 175
   fat-storage 72
fear x, xii, xxxiii, 4, 98, 112
fearlessness 4
feelings x, xiii, xv, xxii, xxiii,
      xxxiii, xxxviii, xliii, xliv,
      xlv, 1, 3, 5, 7, 17, 18, 24,
      34, 54, 61, 71, 74, 77,
      79, 85, 103, 104, 108,
      109, 110, 114, 115, 116,
      118, 119, 120, 121, 124,
      125, 126, 127, 131, 137,
      139, 144, 145, 151, 158
   feelings of unworthiness 3
fermented foods 76
financial situation 120, 121
fizzy 93, 96, 99, 100
focusing xliv, 107, 110,
      131, 136
food cravings xxxvi, xlii, 19,
      32, 38, 67, 68, 69, 73,
      74, 75, 78, 87, 97, 99,
      100, 171, 181
food rules 37
forbidden xxxix, 13, 23, 25,
      141, 149
   forbidden foods 23
forgotten power 3
freedom xii, xxxix, 13, 25, 26,
      91, 98, 136
fried foods 69

friends ix, xii, xxi, xxiv, xxxiii,
    xliv, 2, 25, 50, 56, 105,
    111, 116, 125, 156, 158
frozen meals 45, 69
fructose 78
fruits xiv, xv, xvii, xviii, xxi,
    xxx, 10, 16, 22, 23, 26,
    29, 34, 36, 42, 43, 46,
    47, 48, 54, 64, 69, 71,
    76, 79, 90, 101, 123,
    129, 144, 153, 161, 162,
    173, 174
    fruit-infused water 42, 43
fulfillment 4
fullness xxxii, xli, 15, 17, 55,
    57, 62, 109
functional foods xviii, 176

G

ginger xviii, 28, 29, 33, 36, 39,
    52, 53, 122, 128, 143,
    164, 165, 167, 168, 169,
    176, 177
ginger pear shake 28, 164
gluten 70, 72
gluten-free 70, 72
glycemic index 47
God xxix, xxxvi, 3, 117, 144
grant permission 93, 99
grapefruit 43, 47, 96, 174
gratitude x, 108, 110, 114, 118,
    119, 136
    gratitude journal 119
    gratitude journaling x
greens xvi, xvii, xviii, xxx,
    19, 22, 34, 36, 40, 41,
    47, 48, 58, 80, 81, 90,
    163, 171, 172, 173, 175,
    177, 178
green tea xvi, 34, 177
gut feeling 144, 145, 151
gut health 69, 74, 87
gut-loving chocolate peanut
    butter shake 89, 166

H

habits xxx, xxxv, xxxvii, xlii,
    32, 45, 46, 50, 51, 67,
    77, 84, 88, 97, 132, 151,
    179, 181
    habit xxx, xxxv, xxxvii,
        xlii, 32, 45, 46,
        50, 51, 67, 77, 84,
        88, 97, 132, 151,
        179, 181
hand sanitizers 74, 77
happiness v, 4, 5, 118, 125
hara hachi bu xxi
harmony iii, xiii, xxxvi,
    xxxviii, 6, 51, 89
head hunger
    head-hunger 69, 83, 84,
        86, 88
healing xxxv, 37, 44, 59, 69,
    136, 151
    healing foods 37
health iii, ix, xii, xiii, xiv, xv,
    xvi, xviii, xxv, xxix,
    xxxvi, xxxvii, xxxviii,
    xxxix, xl, xliii, xliv, 2, 3,
    4, 5, 6, 9, 10, 13, 15, 17,
    21, 22, 26, 27, 28, 29,

189

31, 33, 37, 38, 39, 46,
48, 49, 50, 51, 52, 53,
54, 63, 64, 68, 69, 74,
75, 80, 81, 87, 89, 90,
94, 97, 100, 101, 108,
111, 112, 113, 114, 120,
122, 123, 128, 129, 131,
132, 135, 136, 141, 143,
144, 148, 152, 156, 157,
159, 161, 162, 180
healthy choices xliv, xlv,
2, 131, 133, 136,
148, 150
healthy brain shake 63, 165
healthy fat xvi, xvii, 41, 60, 69,
79, 90, 175
healthy protein xvi, xvii, 19, 48
heart disease 44, 49
herbs xv, xviii, 34, 36, 43,
48, 176
Hershey's Kisses 23, 25
Hershey's Kiss 23, 24, 25
higher power 3
higher self ix, x, xxxii, xxxv,
xxxix, xlii, xliv, xlv, 3, 4,
6, 7, 8, 20, 26, 27, 28,
52, 67, 85, 86, 88, 89,
100, 125, 131, 133, 143,
144, 148, 149, 150, 156
honor your cravings 67, 92,
93, 99
honor your craving 67, 92,
93, 99
hope x, xii, 4, 27, 118, 158
hopelessness 4
hormones 72, 78, 87, 112

human body xxxii, 19, 44, 112
hummus 94, 95
hunger xvii, xxi, xxvii, xxxix,
xli, 15, 16, 17, 18, 19,
20, 54, 55, 56, 57, 58,
59, 60, 62, 63, 69, 71,
72, 73, 77, 78, 81, 82,
83, 84, 86, 88
hunger scale 55, 59, 62
hydration 41

I

"I am" statements 124, 127
"I am" xliii, 103, 113, 123,
124, 127, 133
"I am" statement 124, 127
imperfection xlii, 67, 90, 97,
98, 99
imperfection is perfection xlii,
67, 90
inflammation 44, 45, 46,
52, 69
inner balance 69
inner freedom 91
inner harmony iii, xxxvi,
xxxviii
inner journey xlii, 103
inner voice x, xliv, xlv, 131,
138, 144, 145, 146, 147,
150, 151, 158
inspiration 4, 105, 118
insulin 15, 48, 72
intuition 138, 144

J

Jack Canfield 126
Jalaluddin Rumi 108, 181
Joseph Benner 106
Josh Groban 157
journey xii, xiv, xxxix, xli, xlii,
    13, 67, 77, 103, 109, 137,
    151, 158
joy xxxiii, 4, 6, 27, 108, 118
junk food xxiv, xxx, xxxi, 75

K

kale xiv, xvii, xviii, xxx, 33, 36,
    39, 53, 64, 76, 77, 96,
    122, 128, 165, 166, 167,
    168, 172
kefir 76, 89, 90, 166, 178
kimchi 76, 95, 96
kombucha 76, 96
kryptonite food 93, 149
kvass 76

L

lack of sleep 69, 86, 87, 88
law of attraction 106, 107
leafy greens 36, 47, 48, 81, 171
legumes 34, 36, 41, 175
lemon xviii, 22, 33, 42, 64, 96,
    101, 122, 128, 161, 164,
    166, 167, 168, 174
lentils 36, 40, 47, 175
leptin 69, 77, 78, 79, 87, 180
    leptin resistance 69, 77,
        78, 87, 180

Light of Peace 6, 7, 8, 9, 21,
    28, 52, 63, 89, 100, 121,
    125, 128, 142, 143, 147,
    151, 152, 156, 157, 158
lime xviii, 42, 53, 161,
    165, 174
liquid base xvi
liquor 82
liver 28, 82
live with the end in mind xliv,
    131, 132, 138, 142, 147
long-term results 17
loud hunger 56, 57, 62
love v, xiii, xxiii, xxiv, xliii, 3,
    4, 20, 21, 23, 37, 38, 54,
    56, 68, 112, 114, 116,
    118, 125, 128, 133, 134,
    136, 140, 145, 157, 158
low blood sugar xxxii, 56, 81
low-calorie diet 15
low glycemic 47
lunch xxiv, xxix, 38, 39, 62,
    105, 106, 141

M

maca powder xviii, 36, 128,
    168, 178
Maharishi Mahesh Yogi 155
Mahatma Gandhi 5, 123
Make Peace xiv, xliii, 8, 20,
    21, 27, 51, 61, 62, 87,
    99, 103, 110, 120, 127,
    142, 151
mango 22, 53, 164, 165, 174
manifestation 114, 120, 124
    manifesting 35, 117

Marisa Peer 138
Mark Twain 32
Masaru Emoto 114
matcha xviii, 22, 164, 177, 178
MCT oil xvii, 22, 53, 63, 164, 165, 178
meal plans xiv, 2, 18, 35, 39
    meal plan xiv, 2, 18, 35, 39
    meal planning 38, 138, 171
meditation x, xxxv, xliv, xlv, 119, 131, 135, 137, 141, 142, 146, 147, 148, 151
    meditate 85, 147, 148
    meditation apps 148
Melanie's go-to power shake 36, 128, 168
mental exercise 126
Michael Pollan 68
microbiome 74, 75, 77
milk xvi, xix, xxiv, xxx, 9, 22, 28, 53, 63, 89, 100, 122, 128, 143, 152, 163, 164, 165, 166, 167, 168, 169, 177, 178
minerals 43, 68, 73
mirror xxxvi, 90, 110, 123, 133, 137, 157
miso 76
Missing Peaces iii, ix, x, xiv, xv, xxxvi, xxxvii, xxxviii, xxxix, xl, xlii, xliii, xliv, 1, 2, 7, 8, 13, 14, 21, 23, 25, 27, 31, 32, 37, 42, 51, 54, 60, 67, 68, 85, 90, 91, 103, 104, 123, 131, 132, 134, 135, 141, 144, 147, 155, 179, 181, 182
Missing Peace iii, ix, x, xiv, xv, xxxvi, xxxvii, xxxviii, xxxix, xl, xlii, xliii, xliv, 1, 2, 7, 8, 13, 14, 21, 23, 25, 27, 31, 32, 37, 42, 51, 54, 60, 67, 68, 85, 90, 91, 103, 104, 123, 131, 132, 134, 135, 141, 144, 147, 155, 179, 181, 182
moderation 38
mood-boosters xliii, 119, 121
    mood-booster xliii, 119, 121
morning declaration 99
mother 84, 118, 123, 125
must-have foods 32

N

Napoleon Hill 106
National Association of Anorexia Nervosa and Associated Disorders xxxii
National Sleep Foundation 86
natto 76
Nature iv, xxvii, xxxvi, xlv, 3, 6, 20, 32, 37, 68, 80, 91, 114, 119, 140, 144, 145, 147, 148, 149

negative emotions xlv, 4, 7, 121, 125, 127

Neville Goddard 106

no food is forbidden xxxix, 13, 23, 141

non-celiac gluten sensitivity 70
NCGS 70

notebook 127

nutrients xiv, xxix, 15, 19, 34, 38, 52, 60, 69
nutrient-rich foods xiv, 34, 69

nuts xv, xvi, xvii, 19, 25, 26, 34, 36, 41, 47, 69, 70, 71, 76, 77, 79, 89, 96, 106, 166, 175, 176, 178

O

olive oil 19, 41, 48, 79

omelet 34, 39

onion 40, 41, 76, 172

Operation Mood-Booster 119

opioids 73

overeating xxviii, 17, 19, 56, 61, 69, 75

overexercising xxvii, xxviii, 109

P

pancakes 39, 70

parsley 40, 177

passion ix, xxxvi, 4, 174

Path to Peace xxxvii, xxxviii, xxxix, xli, xlii, 8, 13, 67, 103

peace iii, ix, x, xii, xiii, xiv, xv, xvi, xxxiii, xxxvi, xxxvii, xxxviii, xxxix, xl, xli, xlii, xliii, xliv, xlv, 1, 2, 3, 4, 5, 6, 7, 8, 9, 10, 13, 14, 20, 21, 22, 23, 25, 27, 28, 29, 31, 32, 33, 37, 39, 42, 46, 49, 51, 52, 53, 54, 55, 58, 60, 61, 62, 63, 64, 67, 68, 85, 87, 89, 90, 91, 94, 98, 99, 100, 101, 103, 104, 110, 114, 118, 120, 121, 122, 123, 125, 127, 128, 129, 131, 132, 134, 135, 141, 142, 143, 144, 147, 148, 149, 150, 151, 152, 155, 156, 157, 158, 161, 162, 179, 181, 182

Peace of Health xiv, xv, xvi, 9, 10, 22, 28, 29, 33, 39, 52, 53, 54, 63, 64, 89, 90, 100, 101, 122, 123, 128, 129, 143, 144, 152, 161, 162

peaces iii, ix, x, xii, xiii, xiv, xv, xvi, xxxiii, xxxvi, xxxvii, xxxviii, xxxix, xl, xli, xlii, xliii, xliv, xlv, 1, 2, 3, 4, 5, 6, 7, 8, 9, 10, 13, 14, 20, 21, 22, 23, 25, 27, 28, 29, 31, 32, 33, 37, 39, 42, 46,

49, 51, 52, 53, 54,
55, 58, 60, 61, 62,
63, 64, 67, 68, 85,
87, 89, 90, 91, 94,
98, 99, 100, 101,
103, 104, 110, 114,
118, 120, 121, 122,
123, 125, 127, 128,
129, 131, 132, 134,
135, 141, 142, 143,
144, 147, 148, 149,
150, 151, 152, 155,
156, 157, 158, 161,
162, 179, 181, 182
PeaceMeal 38, 39, 40, 52,
60, 171
peaches 143, 169
peachy keen shake 143, 168
peanut butter xxix, xxx, xxxi,
27, 89, 96, 143, 166, 169
pears xvii, 28, 29, 47, 52, 76,
164, 174
pepper 40, 41, 95, 96, 172
peppermint extract xviii, 152,
161, 169, 178
perfect health xxxix, 13, 26,
27, 132, 141
perfection x, xlii, 67, 90
perfectly imperfect xlii, 67, 91,
92, 97, 99
permission iv, xxxix, xl, xlii,
13, 24, 67, 91, 93, 97,
98, 99, 100, 142, 159
pickles 76
Pierce Brown 23
pineapple 43, 53, 165, 174

plan xiv, xlii, 2, 18, 35, 39, 67,
82, 88, 99, 141
positive emotions 4, 118,
121, 125
positive emotion 4, 118,
121, 125
possibilities 114, 135
power of your beliefs 111
prebiotic 76, 77, 181
presence 5, 6, 7, 63
present moment xxxviii, xliv,
1, 6, 7, 8, 89, 106, 128,
131, 142, 147, 151
probiotics 76, 79, 90
probiotic 76, 79, 90
process x, xix, xxiii, xxvii, 21,
44, 46, 55, 57, 72, 78,
82, 110, 113, 114, 116,
117, 148, 162
processed foods 35, 45, 46,
60, 69, 70, 72, 73, 76,
78, 133
processed food 35, 45, 46,
60, 69, 70, 72, 73,
76, 78, 133
processed junk food
xxiv, xxx
product recommendation
list 177
protection 7
protein xvi, xvii, xix, 10, 19,
22, 29, 33, 41, 48, 53,
64, 70, 79, 90, 101, 122,
129, 144, 152, 161, 162,
163, 164, 165, 166, 167,
168, 169, 170, 178

pumpkin seeds xvii, xix, 33, 36, 40, 41, 95, 175, 178
purpose iv, v, xiii, 4, 18, 145, 156, 158

Q

quiet hunger 56, 57, 58, 62
quieting your mind xliv, 131

R

receive xxxix, 8, 13, 117, 133
red X xxxix, 13, 24, 25
relationships xiii, xxiii, xxv, xxvi, xxxvi, 23, 24, 108, 117, 120, 121, 125, 151
release resistance 21, 110, 119
resistance x, xxxix, 13, 14, 21, 69, 77, 78, 87, 110, 119, 138, 139, 180
rest in living peace 155
restoring peace xxxix, xli, xlii, xliii, xlv
return to your roots xl, xli, 31, 54, 55, 62
rituals x, xxii, xxxiii
romantic relationship 120, 121
rope burn exercise 116
Rule of 20 97, 98
rules xxiv, 24, 35, 37, 38, 97, 98, 137, 171

S

saccharin 15, 80
sadness xxxiii, 4, 125

salad xxiv, xxix, 19, 20, 32, 39, 40, 41, 48, 81
salmon 19, 40, 41, 71, 79, 140
salt xix, 60, 68, 69, 72, 73, 91, 93, 94, 95, 162, 178
salty/crunchy 95
sauerkraut 76, 95
the Secret 104, 106
sedentary lifestyle 46
seeds xiv, xv, xvi, xvii, xix, 19, 26, 33, 34, 36, 40, 41, 47, 69, 70, 77, 79, 95, 101, 162, 167, 174, 175, 176, 177, 178
seek no further xxxviii, 1, 2, 21
self-care xliv, 51
self-defeating thoughts xxxvi, xxxviii, 1, 7
self-love xliii, 157
self-talk xlii, xliii, 103, 104
serenity 7
shakes xiv, xv, xvi, xvii, xviii, xix, 9, 10, 22, 23, 28, 29, 33, 36, 39, 52, 53, 54, 63, 64, 89, 90, 95, 100, 101, 122, 123, 128, 129, 143, 144, 152, 153, 161, 162, 163, 164, 165, 166, 167, 168, 169
    berry power shake 100, 167
    chocolate almond cherry shake 9, 163
    chocolate mint shake 152, 169

clean & green shake 22

ginger pear shake 28, 164

gut-loving chocolate
      peanut butter shake
      89, 166

healthy brain shake
      63, 165

Melanie's go-to power
      shake 36, 128, 168

peachy keen shake
      143, 168

strawberry lemon surprise
      shake 122, 167

tropical turmeric shake
      39, 53, 165

Shane Koyczan 90

simplicity 3, 48

skin problems 35

sleep xl, 8, 31, 45, 69, 74, 86,
      87, 88, 115, 180

      sleep-deprived 87

Soren Kierkegaard v

Source v, ix, x, xvi, xxxvi, xlii,
      3, 9, 41, 42, 67, 68, 85,
      87, 88, 89, 91, 117, 118,
      144, 145, 149

spices xv, xviii, 34, 36, 41, 48,
      93, 176

spicy 93, 96, 99, 100

spinach xvii, xviii, 22, 27, 36,
      40, 53, 64, 76, 141, 152,
      164, 165, 166, 169, 173

spiralized 40

Spirit xxxvi, 3, 145

spirituality 108, 120, 121

Steve Jobs 106, 107, 137, 182

stevia 80

stillness xliv

stomach discomfort 35

strawberries 43, 76, 95, 122,
      168, 174

strawberry lemon surprise
      shake 122, 167

stress xxvii, 68, 84, 85, 86,
      112, 148

sucralose xvi, 15, 80

sugars xvi, xix, xxix, xxxi,
      xxxii, 2, 10, 15, 19, 22,
      28, 29, 41, 43, 44, 46,
      47, 48, 53, 56, 60, 64,
      68, 69, 70, 72, 73, 77,
      78, 79, 80, 81, 82, 87,
      90, 91, 95, 101, 111,
      122, 129, 133, 134, 136,
      144, 152, 163, 164, 165,
      166, 167, 168, 169, 170,
      180, 181

      sugar xvi, xix, xxix, xxxi,
      xxxii, 2, 10, 15,
      19, 22, 28, 29, 41,
      43, 44, 46, 47, 48,
      53, 56, 60, 64, 68,
      69, 70, 72, 73, 77,
      78, 79, 80, 81, 82,
      87, 90, 91, 95, 101,
      111, 122, 129, 133,
      134, 136, 144, 152,
      163, 164, 165, 166,
      167, 168, 169, 170,
      180, 181

supplements 76, 79

      supplement 76, 79

surrender 115, 120, 157

sweet xv, xxxii, 10, 15, 16, 22, 25, 29, 33, 45, 54, 64, 73, 80, 90, 91, 93, 95, 99, 100, 101, 123, 129, 144, 152, 161, 173, 180

sweetness xv, 10, 22, 29, 54, 64, 80, 90, 101, 123, 129, 144, 152, 153, 161

sweets xv, xxxii, 10, 15, 16, 22, 25, 29, 33, 45, 54, 64, 73, 80, 90, 91, 93, 95, 99, 100, 101, 123, 129, 144, 152, 161, 173, 180

symptoms 70

T

taking action 111

tempeh 41, 76

Theodore Roethke 54

Thich Nhat Hanh 5

thinking v, xxvi, xxviii, xxxvii, xlii, xliii, xlv, 50, 103, 105, 109, 110, 123, 125, 126, 138, 141, 142, 179

thinness xxvi, xxvii

thoughts xxi, xxii, xxiv, xxv, xxvii, xxx, xxxiii, xxxvi, xxxviii, xlii, xliii, xlv, 1, 5, 7, 16, 23, 24, 25, 27, 50, 67, 68, 94, 103, 104, 105, 106, 107, 108, 109, 110, 113, 114, 116, 118, 120, 121, 122, 123, 124, 125, 126, 127, 134, 135, 137, 138, 139, 145, 147, 156, 157, 158, 181, 182

tobacco 45

tortilla chips 81, 91, 94, 95

toxins 75

traffic light hunger scale 59, 62
    traffic light 58, 59, 62

tropical turmeric shake 39, 53, 165

trusting xxxvii, xl, xli, 31
    trust xxiii, xxxviii, xl, xli, xliv, xlv, 1, 17, 31, 37, 51, 63, 107, 111, 131, 146, 152, 158
    trusting your body xli, 31

turmeric xiv, xviii, 33, 36, 39, 53, 64, 128, 165, 166, 168, 177, 178

U

undesirable states 107

Universe xxxvi, 3, 117

unsupportive cravings xli, xlii, 42, 67, 68, 87, 89, 91
    unsupportive craving xli, xlii, 42, 67, 68, 87, 89, 91

urine 42, 73

US Department of Agriculture's Food Guide Pyramid xxviii

V

vegetables xiv, xxii, 16, 26, 33, 34, 36, 39, 40, 41, 47,

48, 51, 68, 69, 71, 76, 79, 90, 95, 171

visualization xliv, 131, 135, 137, 141, 142, 147

vitamins 43, 68, 148

W

waking 8, 148

walk in nature 119

walnuts xvii, xxx, 19, 36, 39, 40, 48, 64, 165, 176

water xvi, xix, xxi, xl, 27, 31, 41, 42, 43, 60, 68, 73, 76, 77, 81, 82, 94, 96, 111, 114, 181

Wayne Dyer xi, 50, 106

weight gain xvii, xxiv, 15, 17, 78

weight-loss 18, 23

well-being iv, xiii, xxxvi, xxxviii, 1, 2, 3, 4, 6, 8, 9, 21, 74, 87, 89, 151

wellness xlii, 20, 46, 67, 150

what-is land 133

what you feed your body most xv, xl, 27, 31, 32, 51, 79, 134

what you resist, persists xxxix, 13, 14, 17, 18, 20, 25, 85, 141

what you think about, you bring about xliii, 103, 104

white flour 69

whole foods xv, 16, 79

wholesome foods xxxv, xl, xlv, 31, 33, 99

willpower 16, 32, 71, 78, 134

wine 38, 81, 82, 97, 98, 156

worry xxix, 4, 7, 17, 61, 75, 119, 135

Y

Yale University's Prevention Research Center 73

yogurt xxi, xxix, 15, 18, 76, 79, 80

Z

zucchini 40, 173